HUMAN AN
COLORING BOOK

BONES
MEDICAL NOTES

50+ Unique Designs

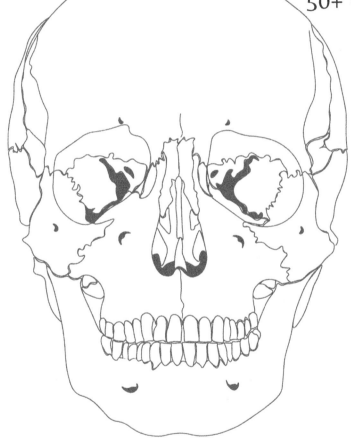

by Delano D. Davis, M.D.

-ANATOMY & PHYSIOLOGY COLORING STUDY GUIDE-

MEDICAL ESSENTIALS +

THE MEDICAL NOTES SERIES

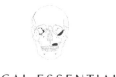

MEDICAL ESSENTIALS +

Illustrated by Delano D. Davis, M.D.
Award Winning Researcher, Tutor, and Medical Illustrator

ISBN: 9798836524371

For questions and customer service;
Send us an email at medicalessentialsplus@gmail.com
Follow Us on Instagram @ medicalessentialsplus
Subscribe to our Youtube channel " Medical Essentials Plus"
for tutorials and Quizzes.

Connect with Us

Scan QR code to visit ➡️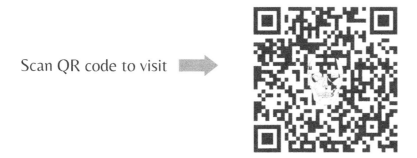

Medical Essentials Plus - Amazon Author Page

Visit our Author page to check out our wide range of atlases, and coloring workbooks on the human anatomy and physiology. We also have beautiful notebooks. Find books on;

- Gross Anatomy and Physiology
- Musculoskeletal System
- Neuroanatomy
- Cardiovascular System Anatomy
- Anatomy notebooks, Journals and more

Scan QR code to visit ➡️

Medical Essentials Plus - YouTube Channel

Visit the medical Essentials Plus Youtube channel and subscribe to get tutorials and quizzes on:

- Gross anatomy and Physiology
- Clinical Medicine
- Clinical Procedures & more

Test your knowledge by taking our quizzes.

Contents

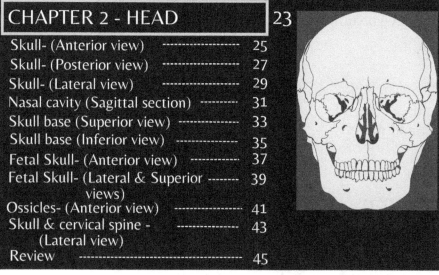
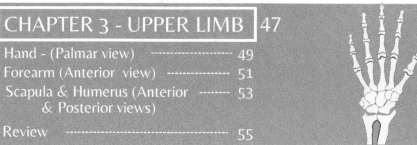
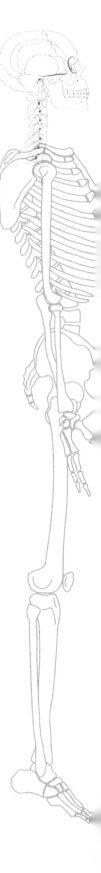

Contents

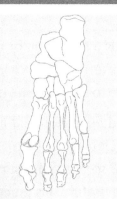
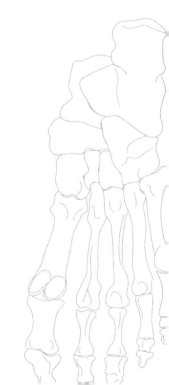

Preface

This book is a collection of unique line drawing diagrams of the human skeleton. It is the digitzed version of sketches done while I was in medical school. It is designed to be used as a supplemental study guide to aid students of anatomy and physiology, and others in the healthcare field.

It should be used to aid in the visual orientation and basic identification of the structures of the human skeleton. From my own experience, learning the human anatomy can present many challenges, so preparing simple line diagrams and coloring them was a good strategy that proved to be quite useful. This practice improved my understanding, retention and recall of core concepts.

The main goal of this book is to help students master the basic configuration of the bones of the human skeleton. No ligaments, muscles, or other attachments have been added. It is the foundation for a series of books that breaks down the human anatomy in a layered manner, with a look at each system individually but not exclusive of each other.

In book two, *"Human Anatomy Coloring book : Muscles"*   a comprehensive overlay of the muscles in relation to the perspective of the bones covered here are presented. For the next step, we recommend getting book two.

Each diagram in this book is labeled with numbers and or letters and structures are identified by using the key list provided. Color coding is done by matching the number or letter of each structure with its corresponding terminology and color swatch in the Key. This will help you to quickly reference each labeled part when reviewing your work. However, there will be structures that cannot be colored in completely, such as bony landmarks, in this case, we recommend the use of a standard color in the swatch, for example. Black, gray, or the same color as the parent bone.

We have included a number of review pages to help promote self-testing. Self-testing promotes content retention and evaluates understanding of the topic covered. Each review page has a diagram that should be labeled and colored, feel free to add your own notes and anotations.

Features:

-Important bony landmarks

-Anatomy flash card style format

-Self-test review pages at the end of each chapter.

-Notes pages

-Mnemonics

-Summaries

-Quick access to our video quizzes, overviews, and tutorials.

Stay tuned for our books on Neuroanatomy, the Musculoskeletal system, the Cardiovascular system, and more. Coloring is an easy and fun way to learn anatomy and physiology. We here at Medical Essentials Plus hope that this book will not only provide entertainment value but also play a valuable role as an educational supplement to the course material of anatomy students everywhere.

Delano D. Davis, M.D.

CHAPTER I

THE SKELETON

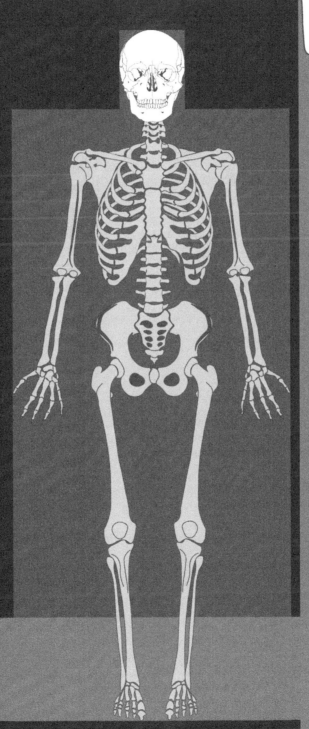

Anatomical Position & Planes

ANATOMICAL POSITION

Sagittal plane

RIGHT LEFT

Coronal plane

SUPERIOR

Transverse plane

INFERIOR

POSTERIOR ANTERIOR

The anatomical position is represented when a subject's body is standing erect, head and eyes are in a forward position, and both arms are at the sides with palms facing forward. The legs are together with the toes pointing forward.

PLANES

Midsagittal or median plane

RIGHT LEFT

Transverse plane (Cross section)

SUPERIOR

INFERIOR

Coronal plane

POSTERIOR ANTERIOR

Skeletal System

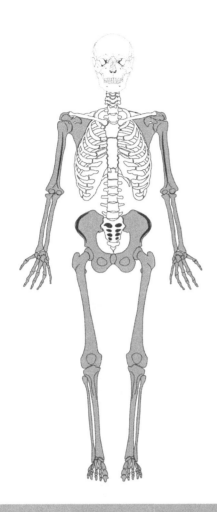

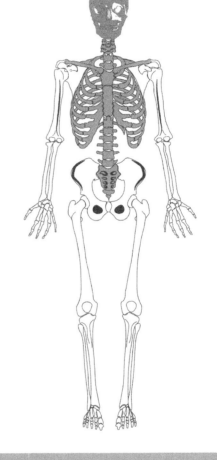

The Appendicular Skeleton is made up of 126 bones:

• Pectoral Girdle - Clavicle (2) & Scapula (2)

• Upper Limb - Humerus (2), Radius (2), Ulna (2), Carpals (16), Metacarpals (10), Phalanges (28)

• Pelvic Girdle - (Innominate, Coxal or Hip bone (2)

• Upper Limb - Femur (2), Patella (2), Tibia (2), Fibula (2), Tarsals (16), Metatarsals (10), Phalanges (28)

The Axial Skeleton is made up of 80 bones:

• Skull - Cranial (8) and Facial bones (14)

• Ossicles (6)

• Hyoid (1)

• Neck - Cervical vertebrae (7)

• Ribcage - Ribs (24), Sternum(1)

• Back - Thoracic vertebrae (12) and lumbar vetebrae (5)

• Sacrum (1) and Coccyx / tailbone (1)

Types of Bones

Types of bones	Examples

Types of bones

- Long bones (90)

Examples

Humerus

others;
- Femur
- Ulna
- Radius
- Tibia
- Fibula

- Flat bones (26)

Scapula

others;

- Sternum
- Cranial bones (Parietal bones)
- Ribs

- Short bones (28)

Carpal bones

Tarsal bones

- Seasamoid bones (4)

Seasamoid bones

- Irregular bones (48)

Vertebrae

others;
- Ossicles
- Hyoid bone
- Hip bones
- Sacrum
- Craniofacial bones (Mandible)

Long Bone Features

Humerus (Partial section)

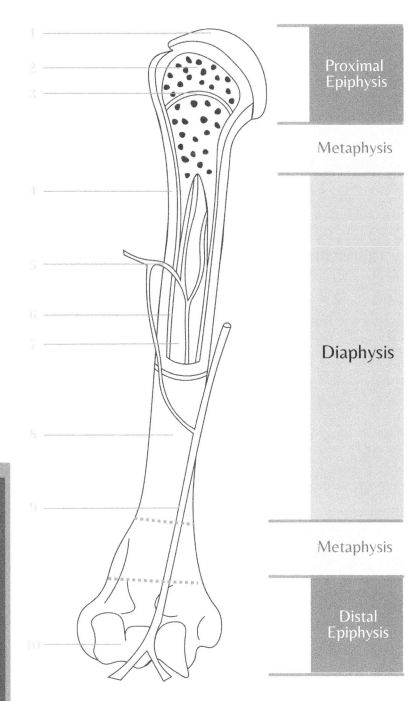

Proximal
Epiphysis

Metaphysis

Diaphysis

Metaphysis

Distal
Epiphysis

1. Articular surface (For Glenoid cavity)

2. Spongy bone (Comprises red bone marrow)

3. Epiphyseal line

4. Compact bone (Hard bone)

5. Artery (Provides nutrients to bone)

6. Endostium (Lining of the Medullary cavity)

7. Medullary cavity (Contains yellow Bone marrow)

8. Periostium (Outermost layer)

9. Brachial artery

10. Articular surface (For Radius and Ulna

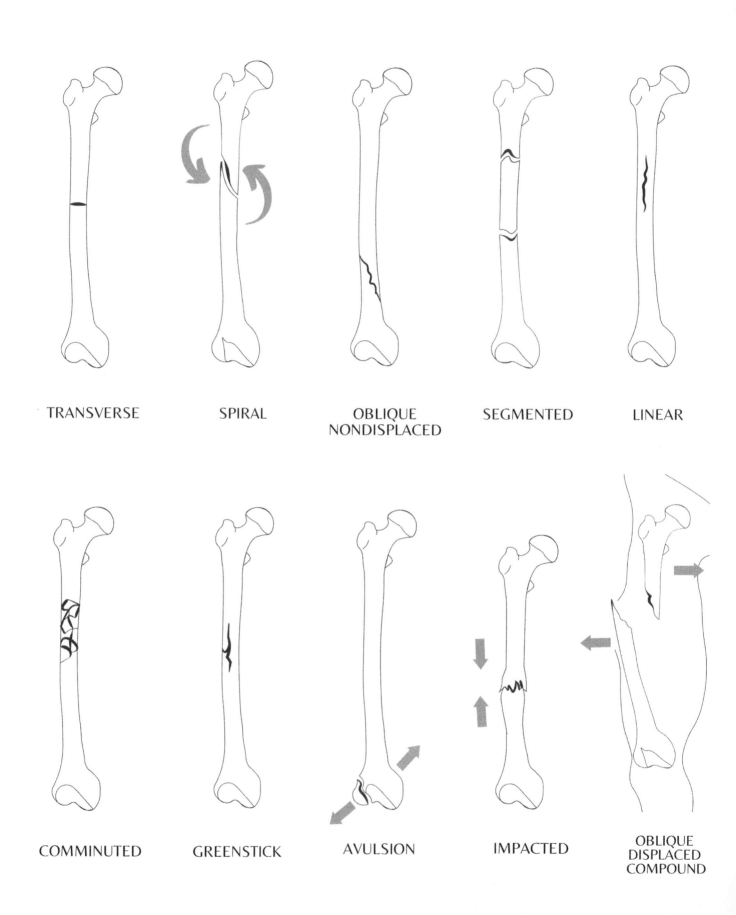

TRANSVERSE

SPIRAL

OBLIQUE
NONDISPLACED

SEGMENTED

LINEAR

COMMINUTED

GREENSTICK

AVULSION

IMPACTED

OBLIQUE
DISPLACED
COMPOUND

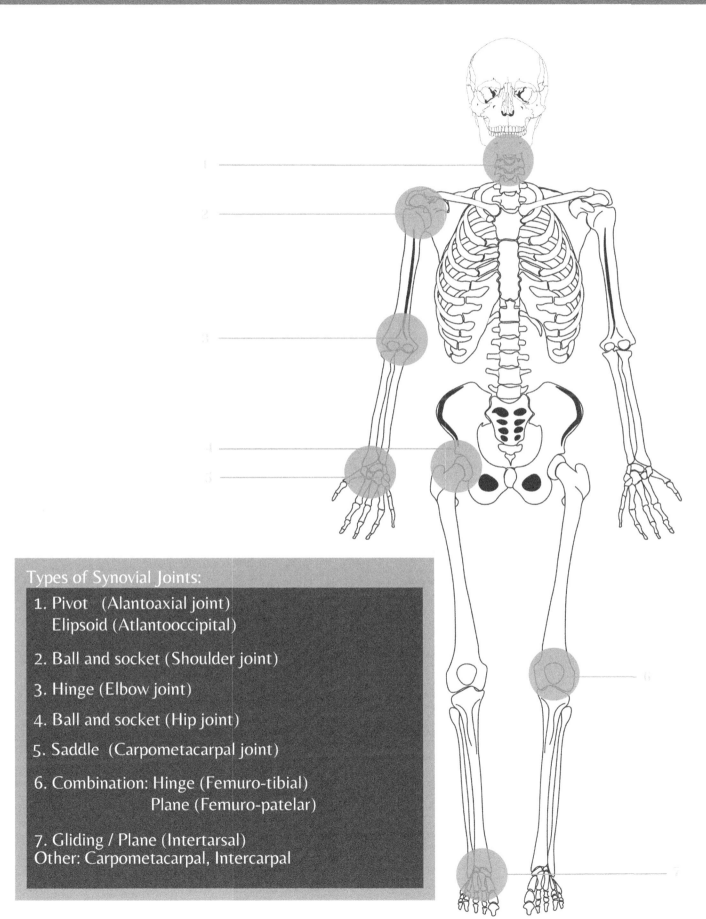

Types of Synovial Joints:

1. Pivot   (Alantoaxial joint)
   Elipsoid (Atlantooccipital)

2. Ball and socket (Shoulder joint)

3. Hinge (Elbow joint)

4. Ball and socket (Hip joint)

5. Saddle (Carpometacarpal joint)

6. Combination: Hinge (Femuro-tibial)
                Plane (Femuro-patelar)

7. Gliding / Plane (Intertarsal)
Other: Carpometacarpal, Intercarpal

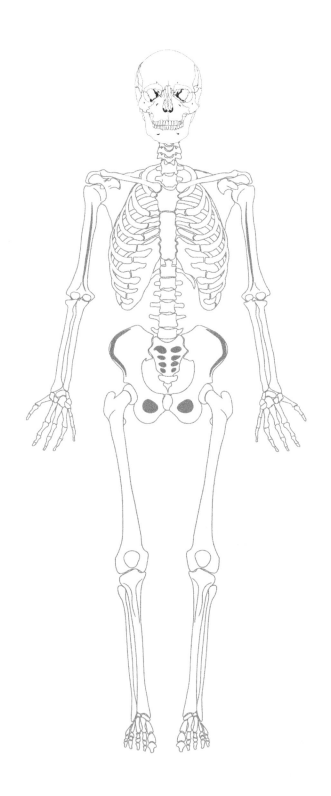

Skeleton (Anterior view)

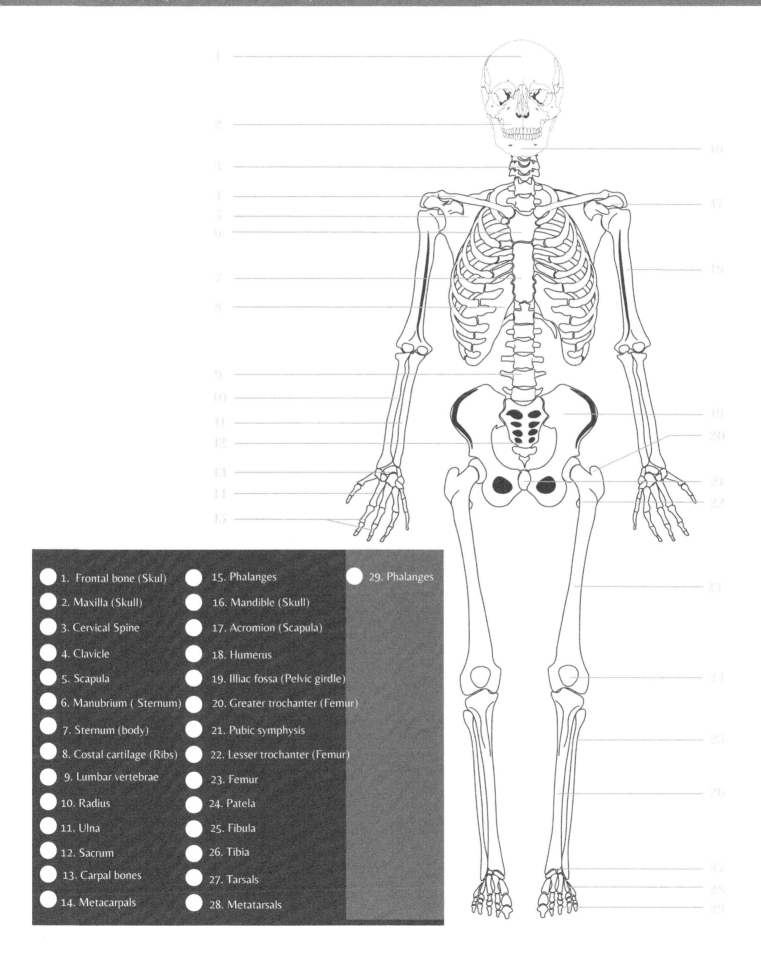

1. Frontal bone (Skul)
2. Maxilla (Skull)
3. Cervical Spine
4. Clavicle
5. Scapula
6. Manubrium (Sternum)
7. Sternum (body)
8. Costal cartilage (Ribs)
9. Lumbar vertebrae
10. Radius
11. Ulna
12. Sacrum
13. Carpal bones
14. Metacarpals
15. Phalanges
16. Mandible (Skull)
17. Acromion (Scapula)
18. Humerus
19. Illiac fossa (Pelvic girdle)
20. Greater trochanter (Femur)
21. Pubic symphysis
22. Lesser trochanter (Femur)
23. Femur
24. Patela
25. Fibula
26. Tibia
27. Tarsals
28. Metatarsals
29. Phalanges

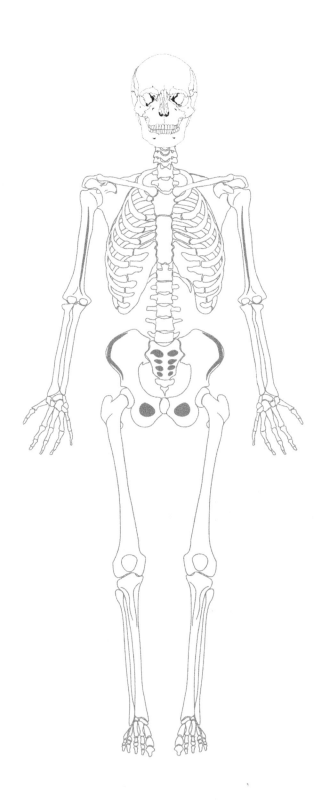

Skeleton (Posterior view)

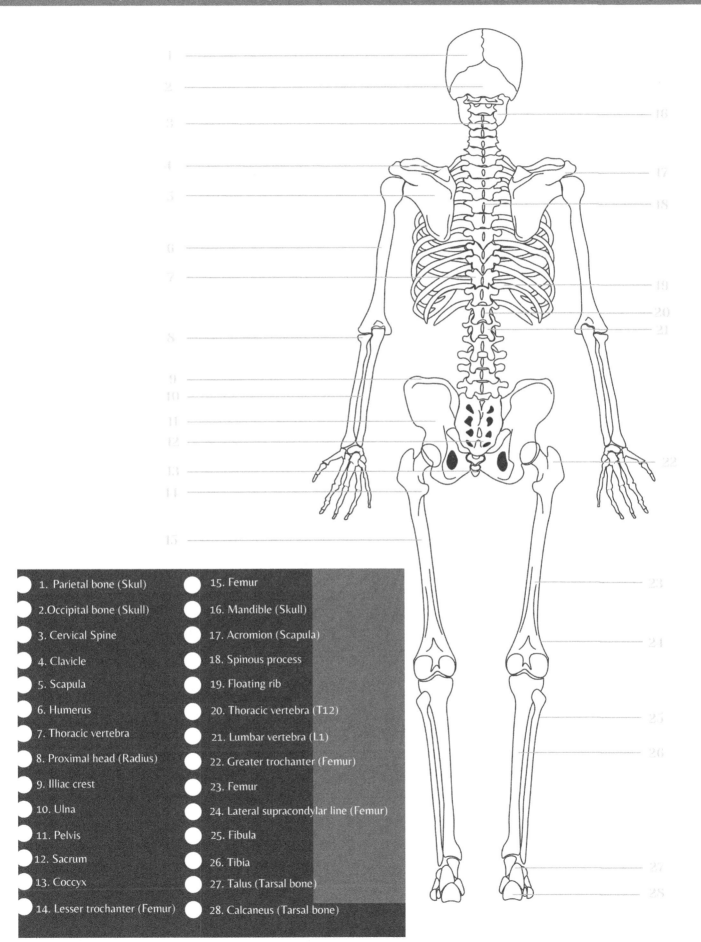

1. Parietal bone (Skul)

2. Occipital bone (Skull)

3. Cervical Spine

4. Clavicle

5. Scapula

6. Humerus

7. Thoracic vertebra

8. Proximal head (Radius)

9. Illiac crest

10. Ulna

11. Pelvis

12. Sacrum

13. Coccyx

14. Lesser trochanter (Femur)

15. Femur

16. Mandible (Skull)

17. Acromion (Scapula)

18. Spinous process

19. Floating rib

20. Thoracic vertebra (T12)

21. Lumbar vertebra (L1)

22. Greater trochanter (Femur)

23. Femur

24. Lateral supracondylar line (Femur)

25. Fibula

26. Tibia

27. Talus (Tarsal bone)

28. Calcaneus (Tarsal bone)

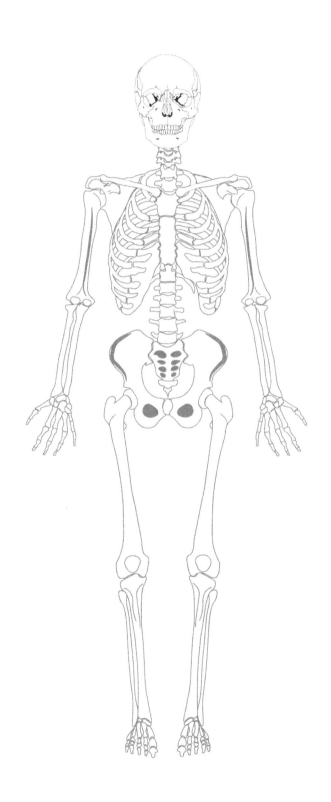

Skeleton (Lateral view)

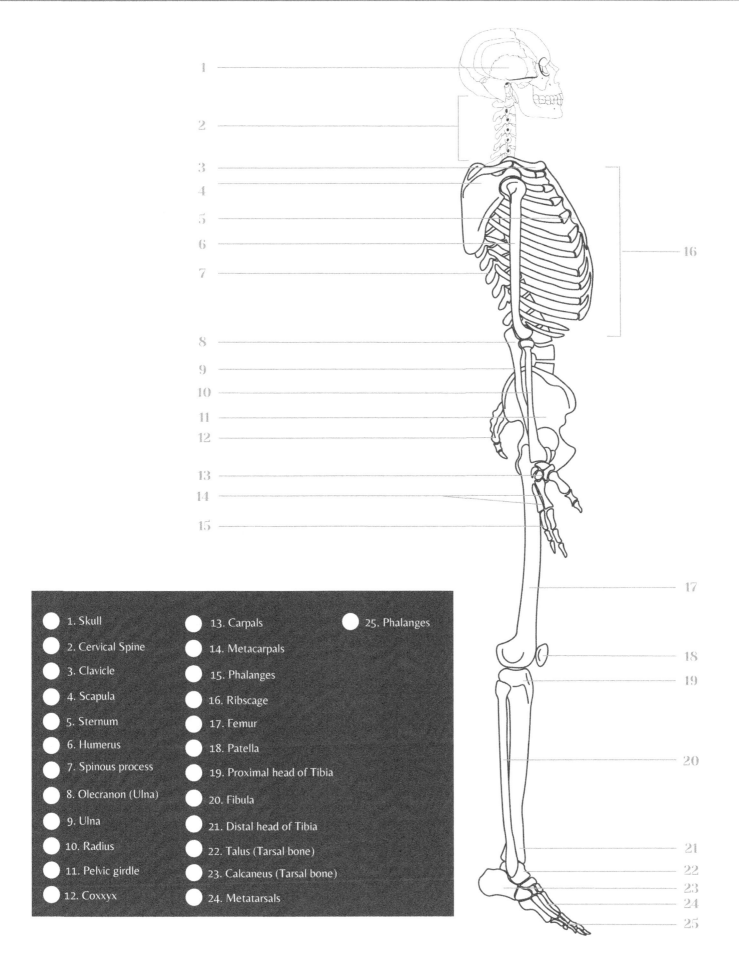

1. Skull
2. Cervical Spine
3. Clavicle
4. Scapula
5. Sternum
6. Humerus
7. Spinous process
8. Olecranon (Ulna)
9. Ulna
10. Radius
11. Pelvic girdle
12. Coxxyx
13. Carpals
14. Metacarpals
15. Phalanges
16. Ribscage
17. Femur
18. Patella
19. Proximal head of Tibia
20. Fibula
21. Distal head of Tibia
22. Talus (Tarsal bone)
23. Calcaneus (Tarsal bone)
24. Metatarsals
25. Phalanges

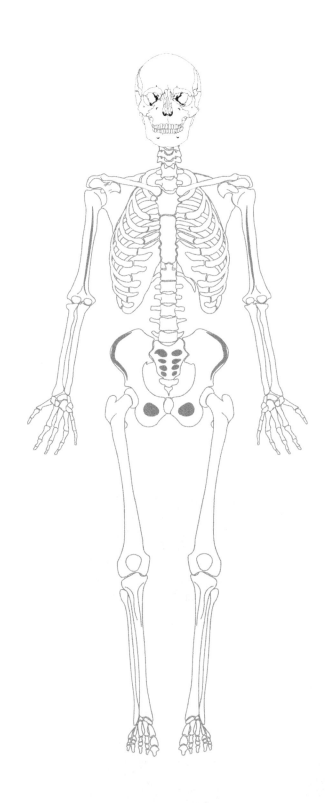

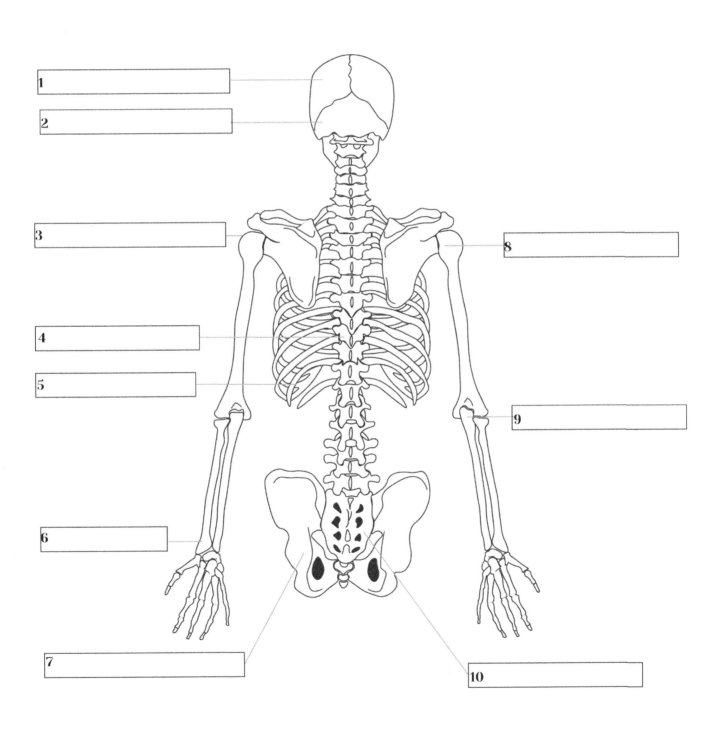

1

2

3

4

5

6

7

8

9

10

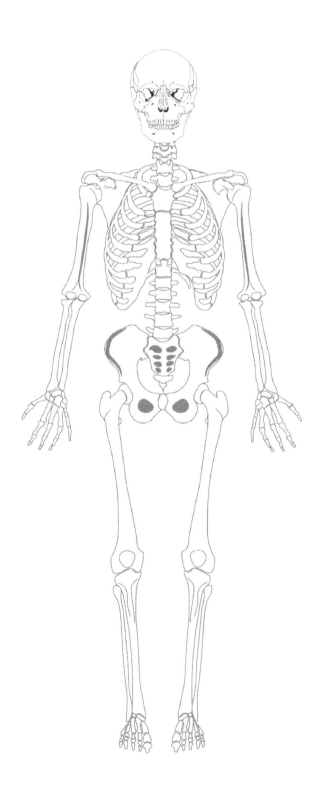

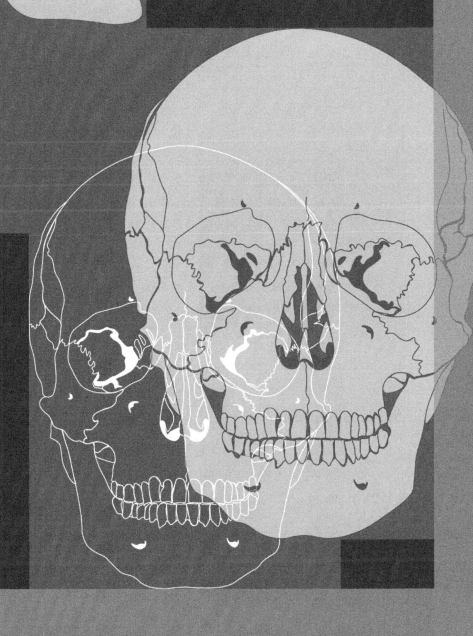

CHAPTER II

HEAD

The Skull

The human skull has 24 bones, eight cranial bones and 14 facial bones. The cranial bones make up the Neurocranium, this is the top and back parts of the skull, it supports and protects the brain.

The eight cranial bones include:

- Two temporal bones (left and right).
- Two parietal bones (left and right).
- One occipital bone.
- One frontal bone.
- One sphenoid bone.
- One ethmoid bone.

The facial bones make up the Viscerocranium or face of the skull and forms the entrance to the eyes, nose, and mouth.

The 14 facial bones include:

- Two zygomatic bones (left and right).
- Two maxilla bones (left and right).
- Two nasal bones (left and right).
- Two Inferior nasal conchae (left and right).
- Two lacrimal bones (left and right).
- Two palatine bones (left and right).
- One vomer.
- One mandible.

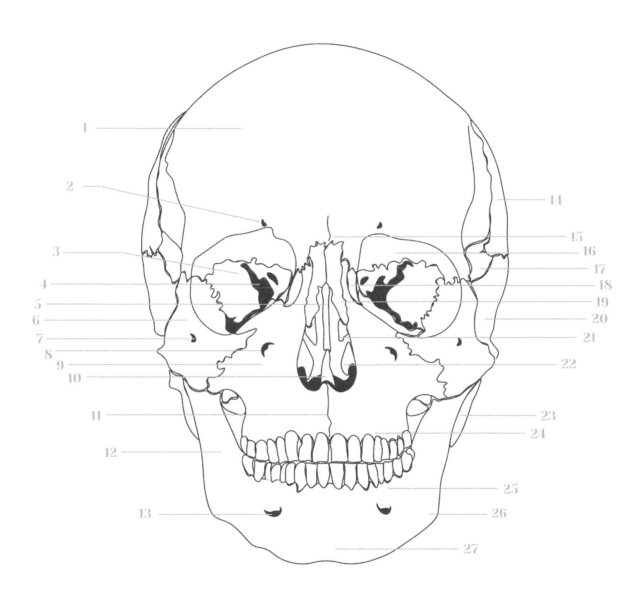

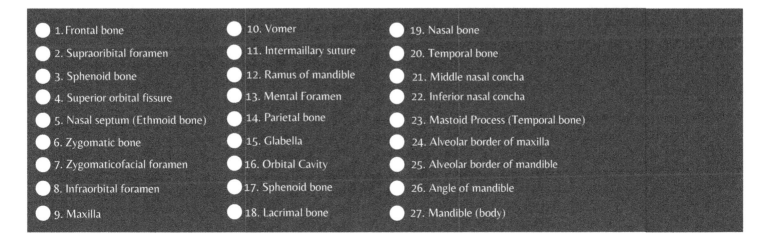

1. Frontal bone
2. Supraoribital foramen
3. Sphenoid bone
4. Superior orbital fissure
5. Nasal septum (Ethmoid bone)
6. Zygomatic bone
7. Zygomaticofacial foramen
8. Infraorbital foramen
9. Maxilla
10. Vomer
11. Intermaillary suture
12. Ramus of mandible
13. Mental Foramen
14. Parietal bone
15. Glabella
16. Orbital Cavity
17. Sphenoid bone
18. Lacrimal bone
19. Nasal bone
20. Temporal bone
21. Middle nasal concha
22. Inferior nasal concha
23. Mastoid Process (Temporal bone)
24. Alveolar border of maxilla
25. Alveolar border of mandible
26. Angle of mandible
27. Mandible (body)

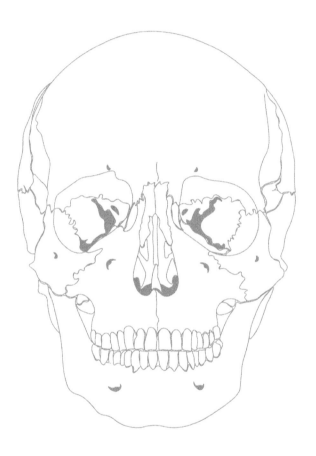

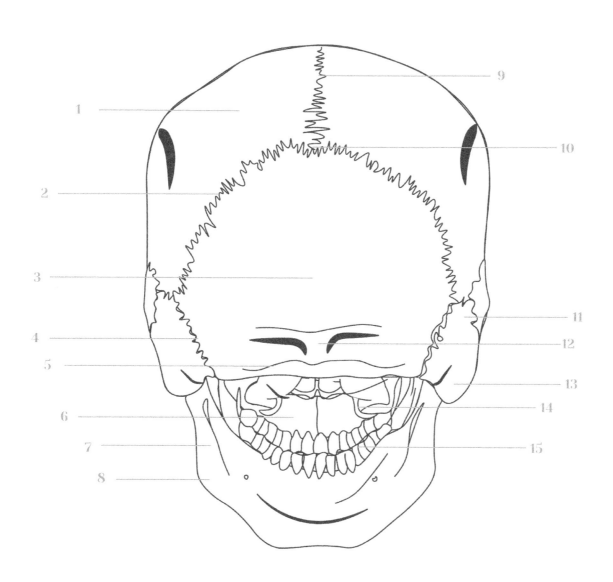

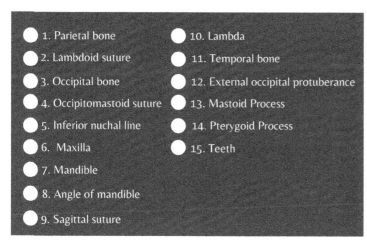

1. Parietal bone
2. Lambdoid suture
3. Occipital bone
4. Occipitomastoid suture
5. Inferior nuchal line
6. Maxilla
7. Mandible
8. Angle of mandible
9. Sagittal suture
10. Lambda
11. Temporal bone
12. External occipital protuberance
13. Mastoid Process
14. Pterygoid Process
15. Teeth

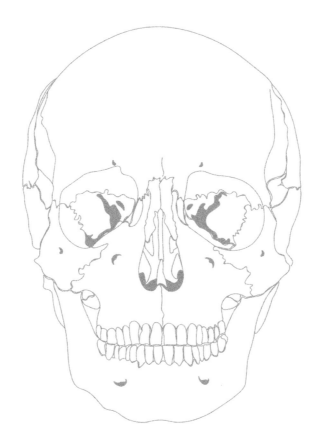

Skull - Lateral view

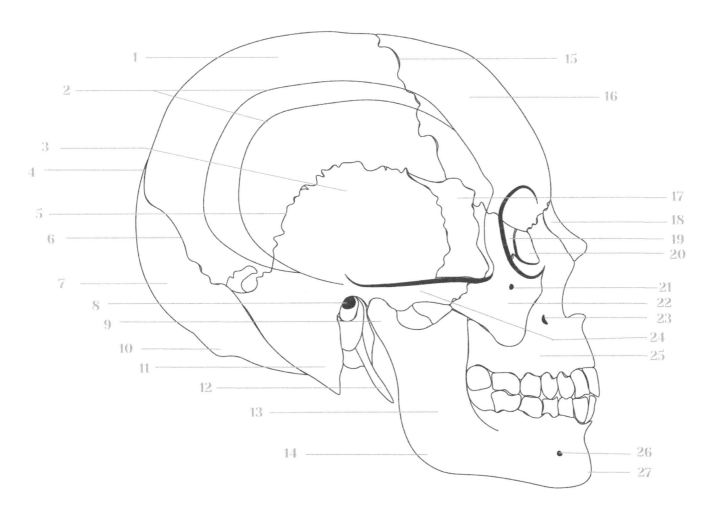

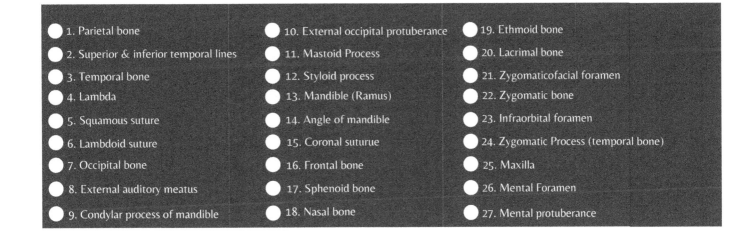

1. Parietal bone
2. Superior & inferior temporal lines
3. Temporal bone
4. Lambda
5. Squamous suture
6. Lambdoid suture
7. Occipital bone
8. External auditory meatus
9. Condylar process of mandible

10. External occipital protuberance
11. Mastoid Process
12. Styloid process
13. Mandible (Ramus)
14. Angle of mandible
15. Coronal suturue
16. Frontal bone
17. Sphenoid bone
18. Nasal bone

19. Ethmoid bone
20. Lacrimal bone
21. Zygomaticofacial foramen
22. Zygomatic bone
23. Infraorbital foramen
24. Zygomatic Process (temporal bone)
25. Maxilla
26. Mental Foramen
27. Mental protuberance

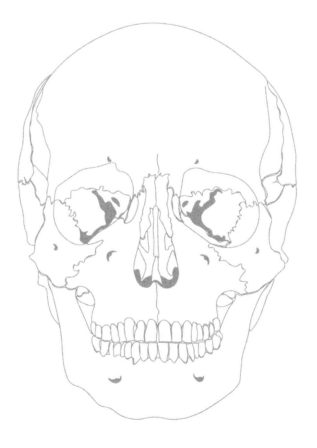

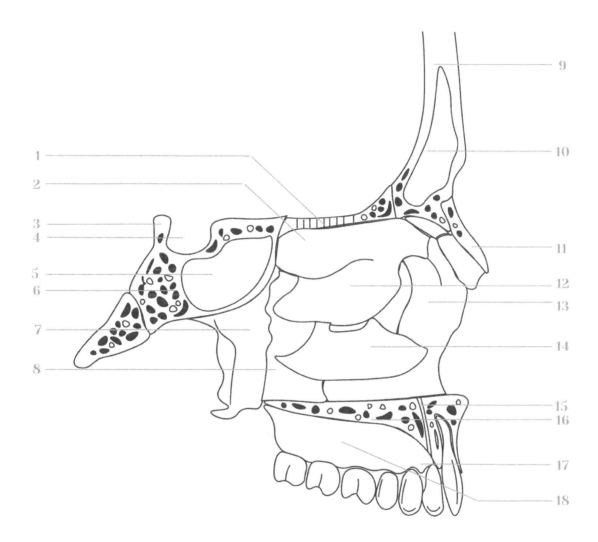

FORAMINA	CONTENTS
2. Cribriform plate (Ethmoid bone)	Olfactory Nerve (Cranial Nerve I)
4. Optic canal	Optic Nerve (Cranial Nerve II) & Ophthalmic artery
19. Superior orbital fissure	Oculomotor Nerve (Cranial Nerve III) Trochlear Nerve (Cranial Nerve IV) Abducens Nerve (Cranial Nerve VI) Ophthalmic Nerve V1 (Trigeminal Cranial Nerve V) Superior ophtalmic vien
20. Foramen Rotundum	Maxillary Nerve V2 (Trigeminal Cranial Nerve V)
6. Foramen ovale	Maxillary Nerve V2 (Trigeminal Cranial Nerve V) Accessory meningeal artery Lesser petrosal nerve
7. Foramen spinosum	Middle meningeal artery & vein Meningeal branch of Mandibular Nerve
9. Internal acoustic meatus	Facial Nerve (Cranial Nerve VII) Vestibulocochlear Nerve (Cranial Nerve VIII) Labyrinthine artery
10. Hypoglossal canal	Hypoglossal Nerve (Cranial Nerve XII)
23. Foramen laserum	Greater Petrosal nerve
24. Carotid canal	Internal Carotid artery & Nerve Plexus
26. Jugular canal	Glossopharyngeal Nerve (Cranial Nerve IX) Vagus Nerve (Cranial Nerve X) Spinal Accessory Nerve (Cranial Nerve XI) Posterior meningeal artery Sigmoid Sinus
27. Foramen Magnum	Medulla Oblongata Vertbral artery Spinal Roots of Spinal Accessory Nerve (Cranial Nerve XI)

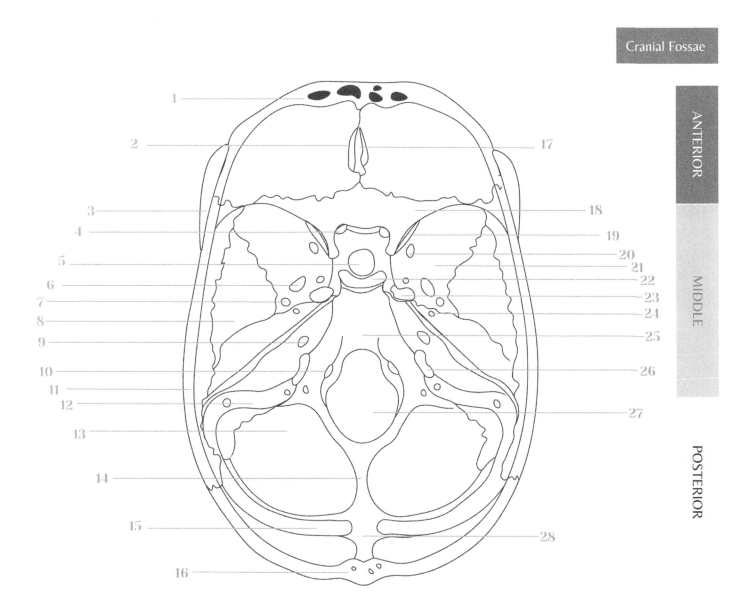

Cranial Fossae

ANTERIOR

MIDDLE

POSTERIOR

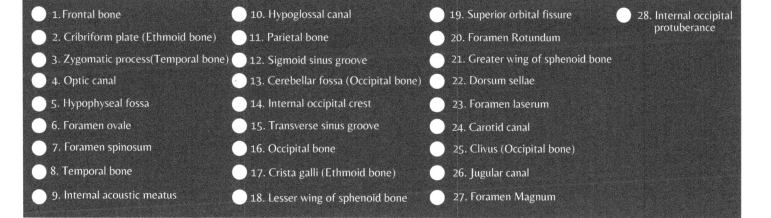

1. Frontal bone
2. Cribriform plate (Ethmoid bone)
3. Zygomatic process(Temporal bone)
4. Optic canal
5. Hypophyseal fossa
6. Foramen ovale
7. Foramen spinosum
8. Temporal bone
9. Internal acoustic meatus

10. Hypoglossal canal
11. Parietal bone
12. Sigmoid sinus groove
13. Cerebellar fossa (Occipital bone)
14. Internal occipital crest
15. Transverse sinus groove
16. Occipital bone
17. Crista galli (Ethmoid bone)
18. Lesser wing of sphenoid bone

19. Superior orbital fissure
20. Foramen Rotundum
21. Greater wing of sphenoid bone
22. Dorsum sellae
23. Foramen laserum
24. Carotid canal
25. Clivus (Occipital bone)
26. Jugular canal
27. Foramen Magnum

28. Internal occipital protuberance

Basilar Skull Fractures

Causes

- Blunt force trauma
- Penetrating injuries
- Falls

Location/ Fossa

● Anterior fossa

● Middle fossa

● Posterior fossa

Signs & Symptoms

- Halo sign
- Racoon eyes
- Eyes movement deficits
- Partial and / or complete loss of vision and sense of smell

- Battle sign
- Hearing loss
- Possible Carotid artery injury
- Balance impairment

- Cranial Nerve injury
- Cervical spine injury
- Vertebral artery injury

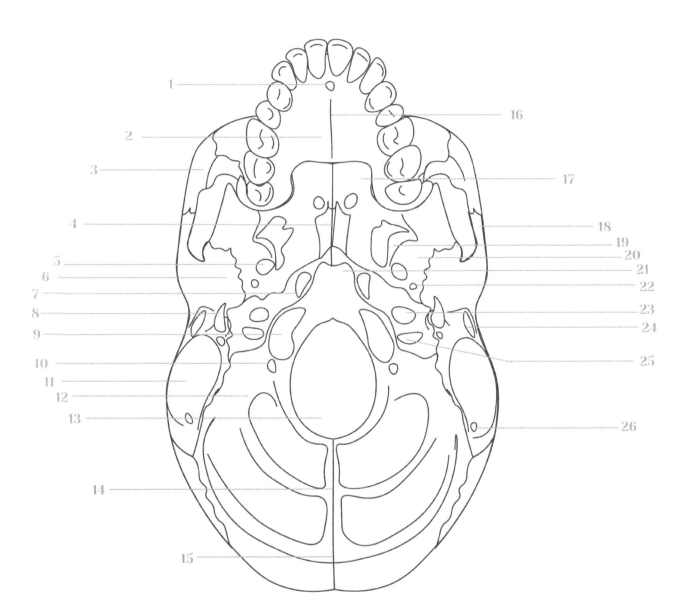

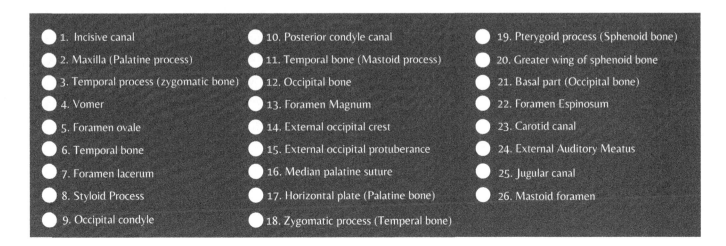

1. Incisive canal
2. Maxilla (Palatine process)
3. Temporal process (zygomatic bone)
4. Vomer
5. Foramen ovale
6. Temporal bone
7. Foramen lacerum
8. Styloid Process
9. Occipital condyle

10. Posterior condyle canal
11. Temporal bone (Mastoid process)
12. Occipital bone
13. Foramen Magnum
14. External occipital crest
15. External occipital protuberance
16. Median palatine suture
17. Horizontal plate (Palatine bone)
18. Zygomatic process (Temperal bone)

19. Pterygoid process (Sphenoid bone)
20. Greater wing of sphenoid bone
21. Basal part (Occipital bone)
22. Foramen Espinosum
23. Carotid canal
24. External Auditory Meatus
25. Jugular canal
26. Mastoid foramen

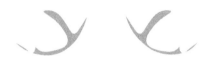

Anterior fontanelle

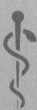

- Diamond shaped

- Usually Measures 1 inch across

- Anterior Fontanelle should be closed by 18 -24 months

- Closure at birth is caused by molding or Microcephaly

- Early closure is called Craniosynostosis as a result of premature closure (Causes vary)

- A sunken fontanelle may be a sign of dehydration and bulging or tense due to increased ICP (Intracranial Pressure).

Posterior fontanelle

Closes at 2- 3 months

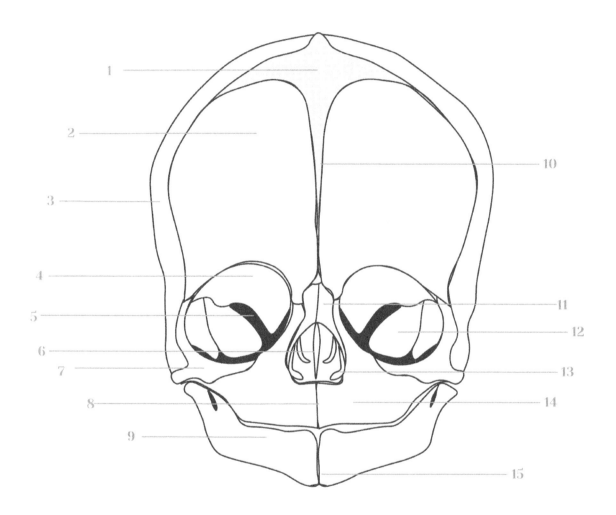

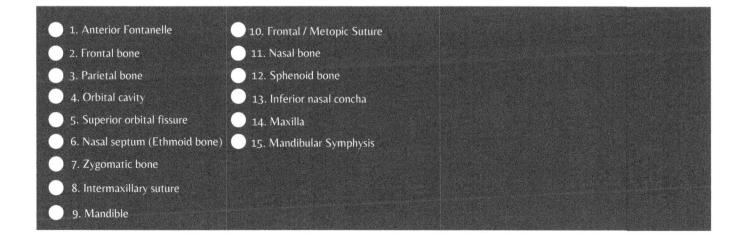

1. Anterior Fontanelle
2. Frontal bone
3. Parietal bone
4. Orbital cavity
5. Superior orbital fissure
6. Nasal septum (Ethmoid bone)
7. Zygomatic bone
8. Intermaxillary suture
9. Mandible
10. Frontal / Metopic Suture
11. Nasal bone
12. Sphenoid bone
13. Inferior nasal concha
14. Maxilla
15. Mandibular Symphysis

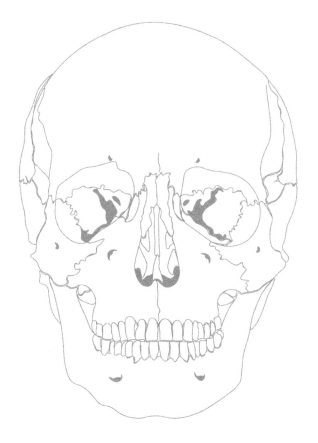

Fetal Skull - Lateral & Superior views

Lateral view

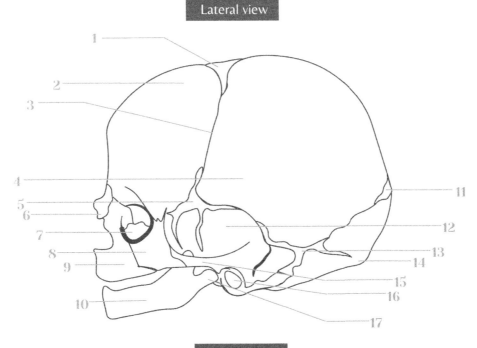

Superior view

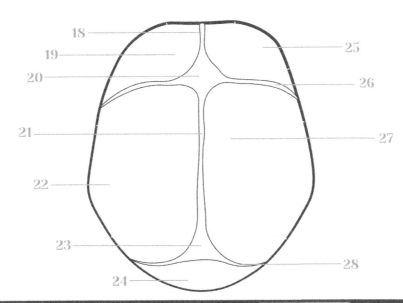

Lateral view

- 1. Anterior fontanelle/ Bregma
- 2. Frontal bone
- 3. Coronal suture
- 4. Parietal bone
- 5. Sphenoidal fontanelle
- 6. Nasal bone
- 7. Orbital cavity
- 8. Zygomatic bone
- 9. Maxilla
- 10. Mandible
- 11. Posterior fontanelle
- 12. Temporal bone
- 13. Mastoidal fontanelle
- 14. External occipital protuberance
- 15. Zygomatic process
- 16. External acoustic meatus
- 17. Condylar process of mandible

Superior view

- 18. Frontal / Metopic suture
- 19. Frontal bone
- 20. Anterior fontanelle/ Bregma
- 21. Sagittal suture
- 22. Parietal eminence
- 23. Posterior fontanelle
- 24. Occipital bone
- 25. Frontal eminence
- 26. Coronal suture
- 27. Parietal bone
- 28. Lambdoid suture

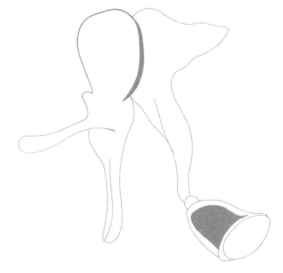

The Ear

The auditory ossicles are the smallest bones in the human body. The function of the ossicle bones is to transfer vibrations from the tympanic membrane (eardrum) to the inner ear. This stimulus is processed and is later sent as nerve impulses via the 8th cranial nerve (VIII) Vestibulocochlear nerve to the auditory center in the temporal lobe.

The middle ear bones include:

-Two (2) malleus bones (one in each ear).
-Two (2) incus bones (one in each ear).
-Two (2) stapes bones (one in each ear).

Ossicles - Anterior view

EXTERNAL EAR   MIDDLE EAR   **INTERNAL EAR**

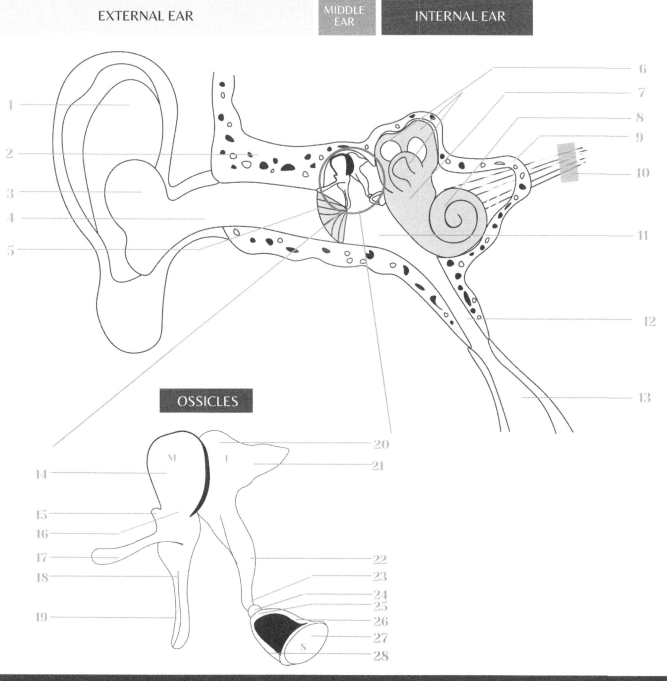

OSSICLES

⚪ 1. Pinna (Auricle)	⚪ 10. Vestibulococlear Nerve (Cranial Nerve VIII)
⚪ 2. Temporal bone	⚪ 11. Tympanic cavity
⚪ 3. Concha	⚪ 12. Auditory tube (Bony part)
⚪ 4. Audtitory canal	⚪ 13. Auditory tube (Cartilaginous part)
⚪ 5. Tympanic membrane	MALLEUS
⚪ 6. Semicircular canals	⚪ M. Malleus
⚪ 7. Bony Labyrinth	⚪ 14. Head (Malleus)
⚪ 8. Cochlea	⚪ 15. Lateral Process (Malleus)
⚪ 9. Internal Acoustic meatus	⚪ 16. Neck

⚪ 17. Anterior Process (Malleus)	STAPES
⚪ 18. Manubrium	⚪ S. Stapes
⚪ 19. Umbo	⚪ 24. Head
INCUS	⚪ 25. Neck
⚪ I. Incus	⚪ 26. Anterior cruz
⚪ 20. Body	⚪ 27. Base (Foot plate)
⚪ 21. Short process	⚪ 28. Posterior cruz
⚪ 22. Long process	
⚪ 23. Lenticular process	

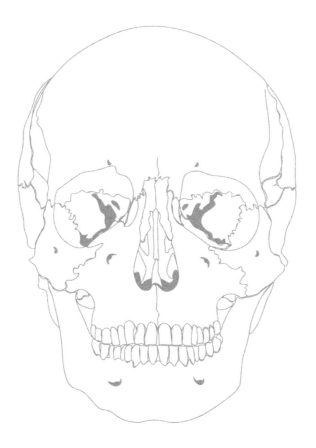

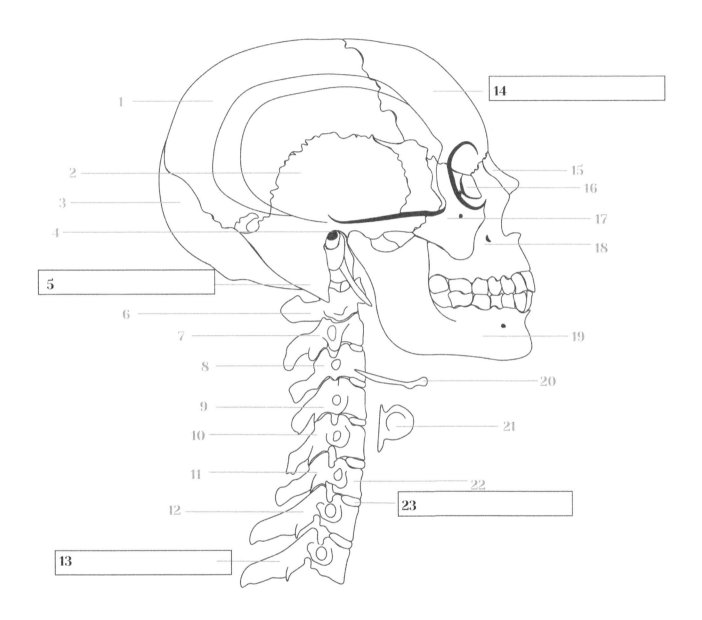

1
2
3
4

| 5 |

6
7
8
9
10
11
12

| 13 |

| 14 |

15
16
17
18
19
20
21
22

| 23 |

Scan me

Test yourself, take the
skull anatomy video
quiz and let us know
your score.

Skull Anatomy Video Quiz

Skull - Review

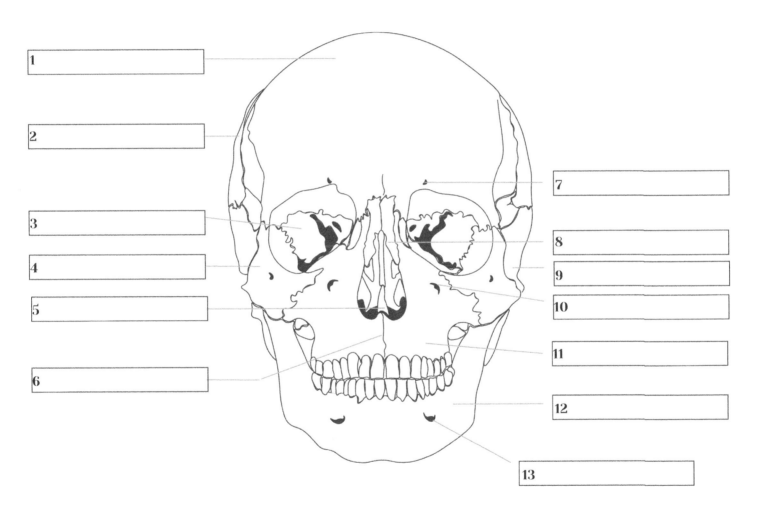

1

2

3

4

5

6

7

8

9

10

11

12

13

1. Frontal bone
2. Parietal bone
3. Sphenoid bone
4. Zygomatic bone
5. Nasal septum (Vomer)
6. Intermaxillary suture
7. Supraoribital foramen
8. Nasal bone
9. Temporal bone
10. Infraorbital foramen
11. Maxilla
12. Mandible (body)
13. Mental Foramen

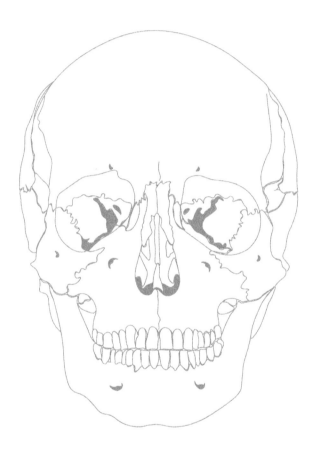

CHAPTER III

UPPER LIMB

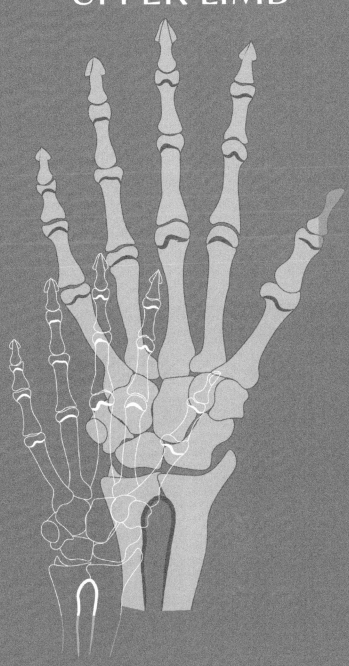

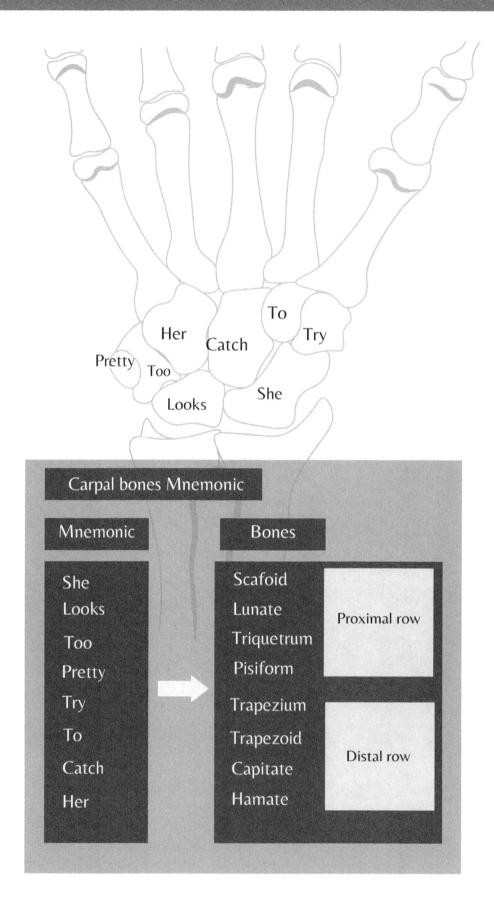

Her
To
Catch
Try
Pretty
Too
She
Looks

Carpal bones Mnemonic

Mnemonic		Bones	
She		Scafoid	
Looks		Lunate	Proximal row
Too		Triquetrum	
Pretty	→	Pisiform	
Try		Trapezium	
To		Trapezoid	Distal row
Catch		Capitate	
Her		Hamate	

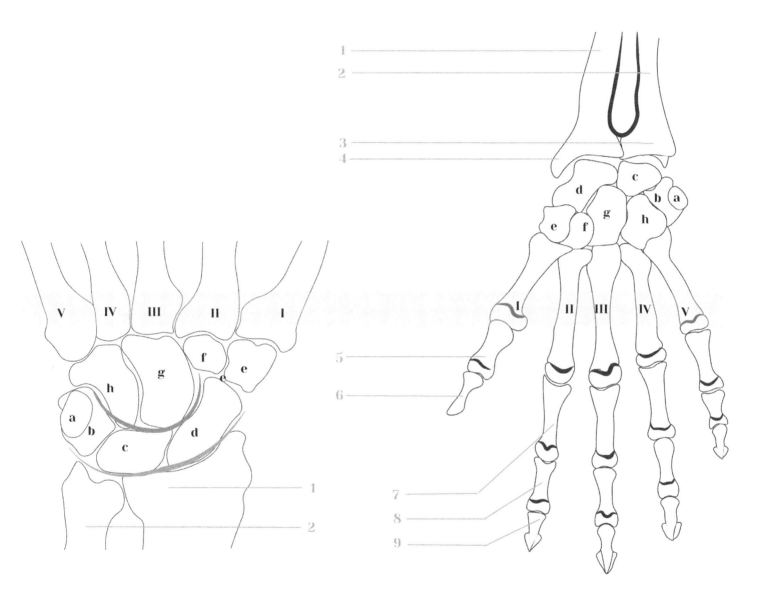

8 Carpal bones

- a. Pisiform
- b. Triquetrum
- c. Lunate
- d. Scafoid
- e. Trapezium
- f. Trapezoid
- g. Capitate
- h. Hamate

5 Metacarpal bones

- (I) 1st Metacarpal bone
- (II) 2nd Metacarpal
- (III) 3rd Metacarpal
- (IV) 4th Metacarpal
- (V) 5th Metacarpal

- 1. Radius
- 2. Ulna
- 3. Distal head of Ulna
- 4. Styloid Process (Radius)
- 5. Proximal phalanx (I)

- 6. Distal phalanx (I)
- 7. Proximal phalanx (II)
- 8. Middle phalanx (II)
- 9. Distal phalanx (II)

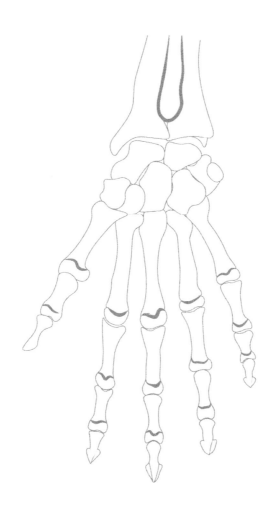

Right Forearm - Anterior view

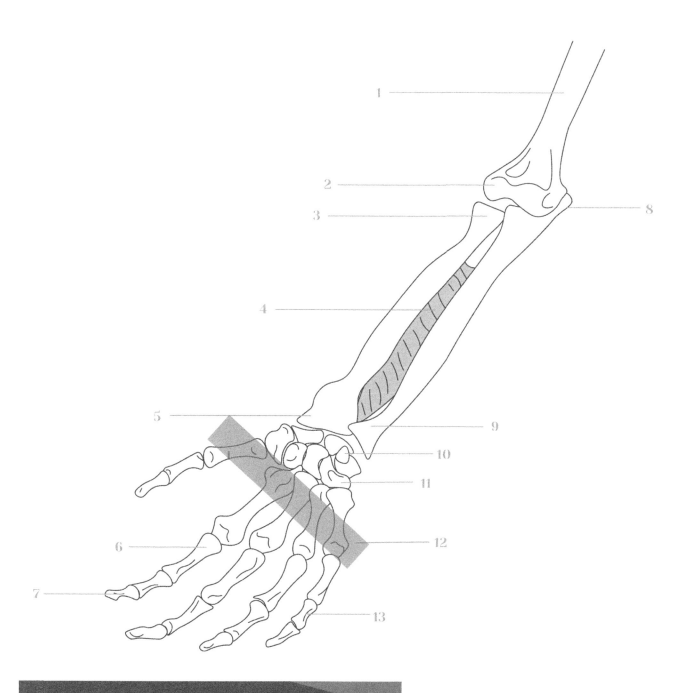

1
2
3
4
5
6
7
8
9
10
11
12
13

1. Humerus
2. Articular Surface
3. Proximal radius
4. Interosseous membrane
5. Styloid Process (Radius)
6. Proximal phalanx
7. Distal phalanx
8. Olecranon (Elbow)
9. Distal head of Ulna
10. Pisiform
11. Hamate
12. Metacarpal bones (x5)
13. Middle phalanx

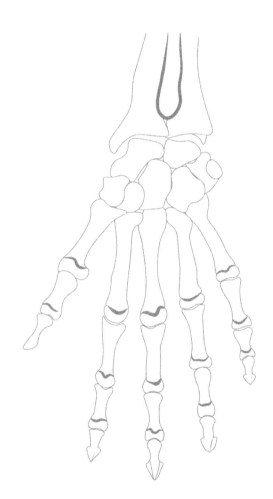

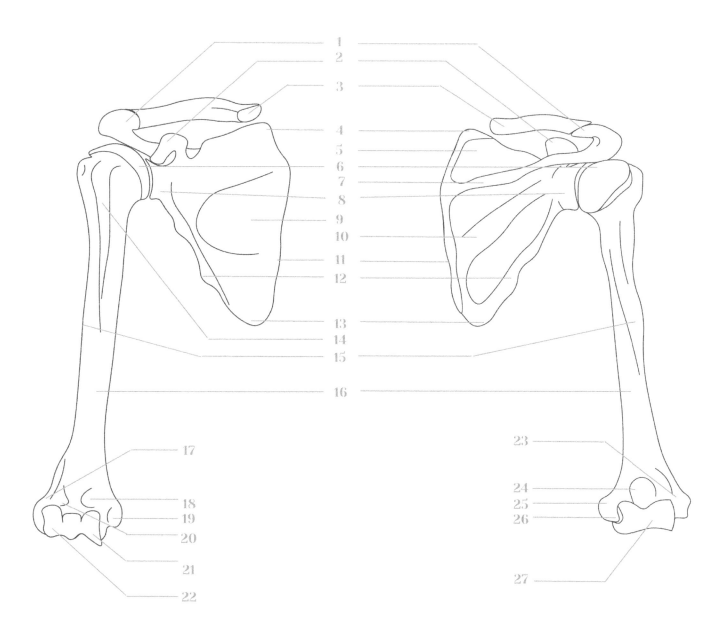

1
2
3
4
5
6
7
8
9
10
11
12
13
14
15
16
17
18
19
20
21
22
23
24
25
26
27

1. Acromion
2. Coronoid process
3. Clavicle (Cut)
4. Superior angle
5. Supraspinous fossa
6. Head of Humerus
7. Spine of scapula
8. Glenoid cavity
9. Subscapula fossa
10. Infraspinous fossa
11. Medial border
12. Lateral border
13. Inferior angle
14. Intertubercular sulcus
15. Deltoid tuberosity
16. Humerus (Shaft)
17. Lateral epicondyle
18. Coronoid fossa
19. Medial epicondyle
20. Radial fossa
21. Trochlea
22. Capitulum
23. Lateral epicondyle
24. Olecranon fossa (humerus)
25. Medial epicondyle
26. Groove for Ulna nerve
27. Trochlea (humerus)

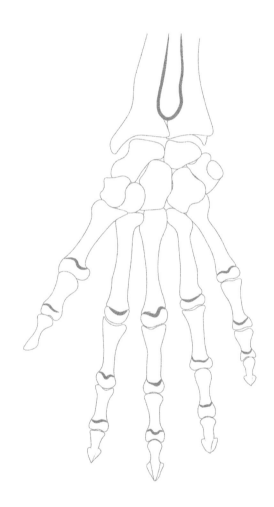

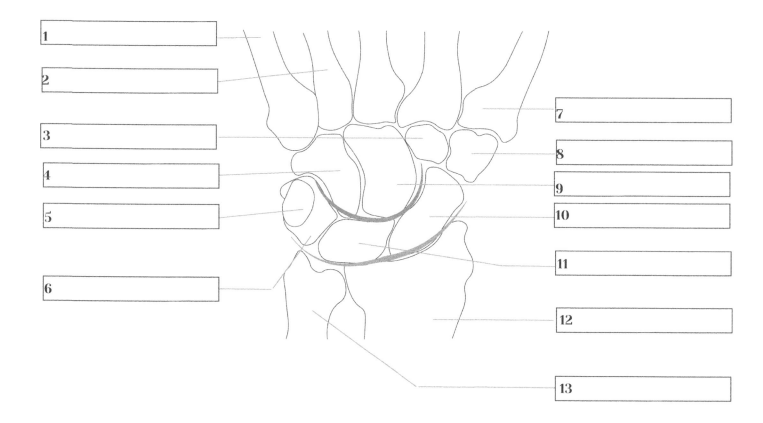

1	
2	
3	
4	
5	
6	
7	
8	
9	
10	
11	
12	
13	

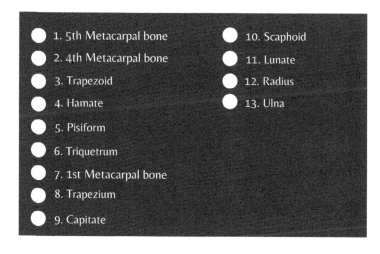

1. 5th Metacarpal bone
2. 4th Metacarpal bone
3. Trapezoid
4. Hamate
5. Pisiform
6. Triquetrum
7. 1st Metacarpal bone
8. Trapezium
9. Capitate
10. Scaphoid
11. Lunate
12. Radius
13. Ulna

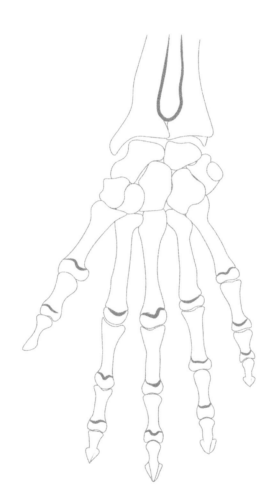

CHAPTER IV

THORAX

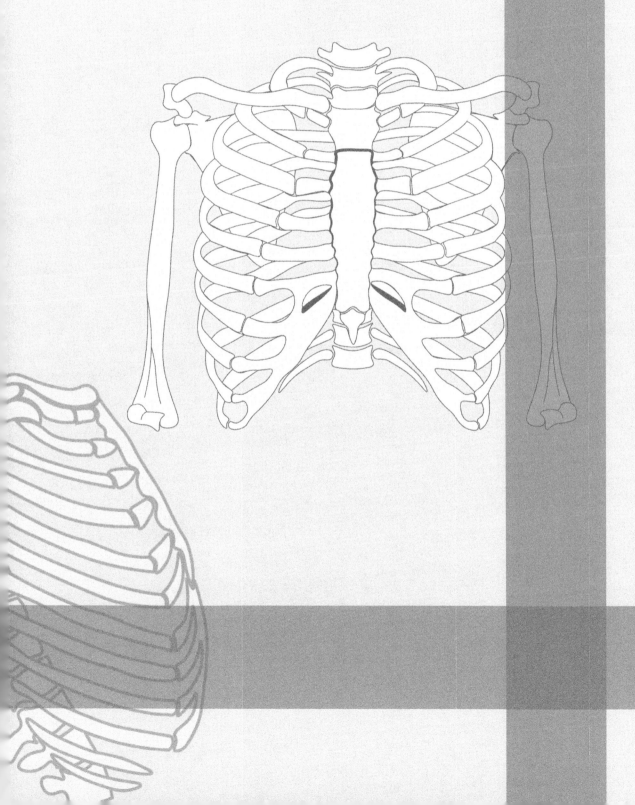

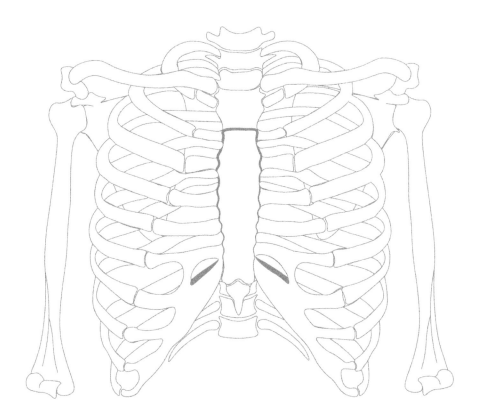

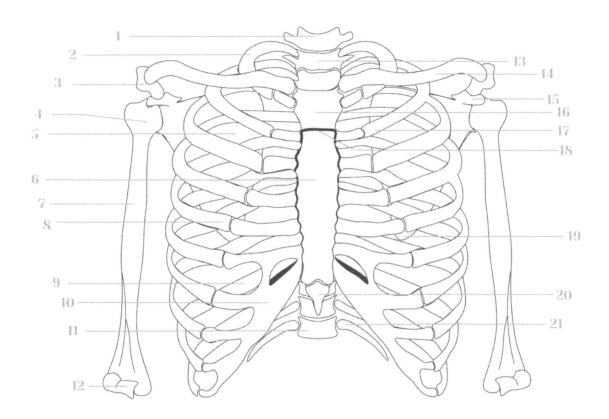

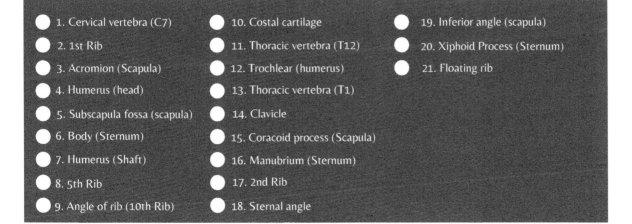

1. Cervical vertebra (C7)
2. 1st Rib
3. Acromion (Scapula)
4. Humerus (head)
5. Subscapula fossa (scapula)
6. Body (Sternum)
7. Humerus (Shaft)
8. 5th Rib
9. Angle of rib (10th Rib)

10. Costal cartilage
11. Thoracic vertebra (T12)
12. Trochlear (humerus)
13. Thoracic vertebra (T1)
14. Clavicle
15. Coracoid process (Scapula)
16. Manubrium (Sternum)
17. 2nd Rib
18. Sternal angle

19. Inferior angle (scapula)
20. Xiphoid Process (Sternum)
21. Floating rib

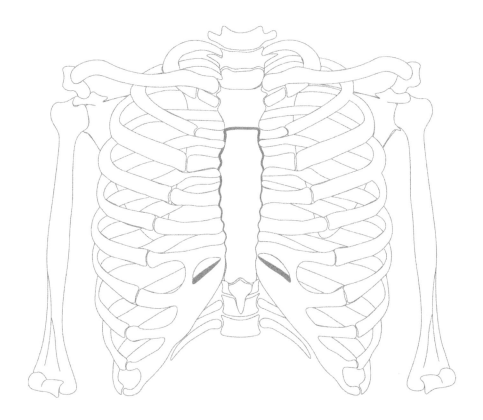

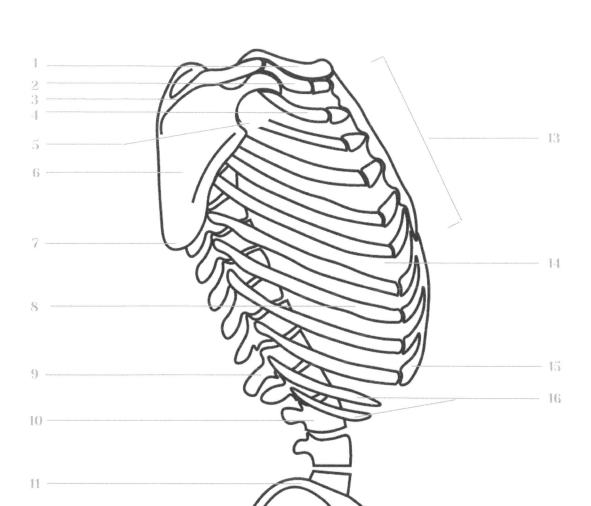

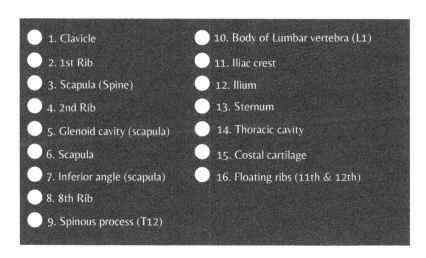

1. Clavicle
2. 1st Rib
3. Scapula (Spine)
4. 2nd Rib
5. Glenoid cavity (scapula)
6. Scapula
7. Inferior angle (scapula)
8. 8th Rib
9. Spinous process (T12)

10. Body of Lumbar vertebra (L1)
11. Iliac crest
12. Ilium
13. Sternum
14. Thoracic cavity
15. Costal cartilage
16. Floating ribs (11th & 12th)

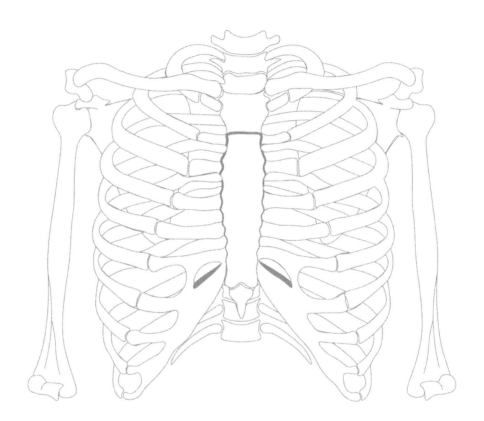

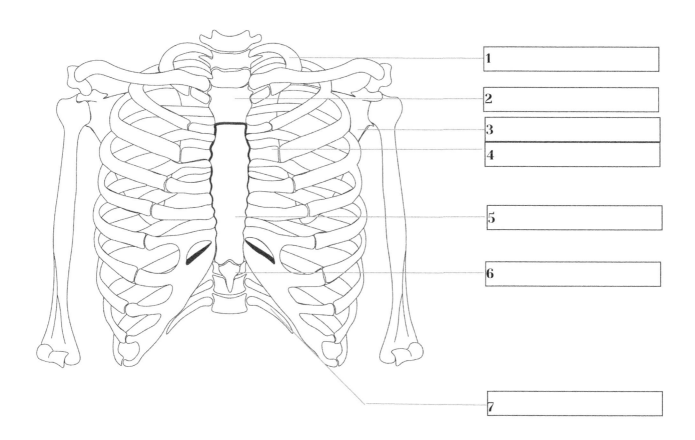

1

2

3

4

5

6

7

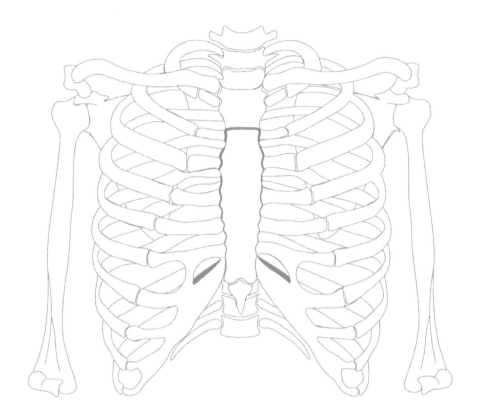

CHAPTER V

LOWER LIMB

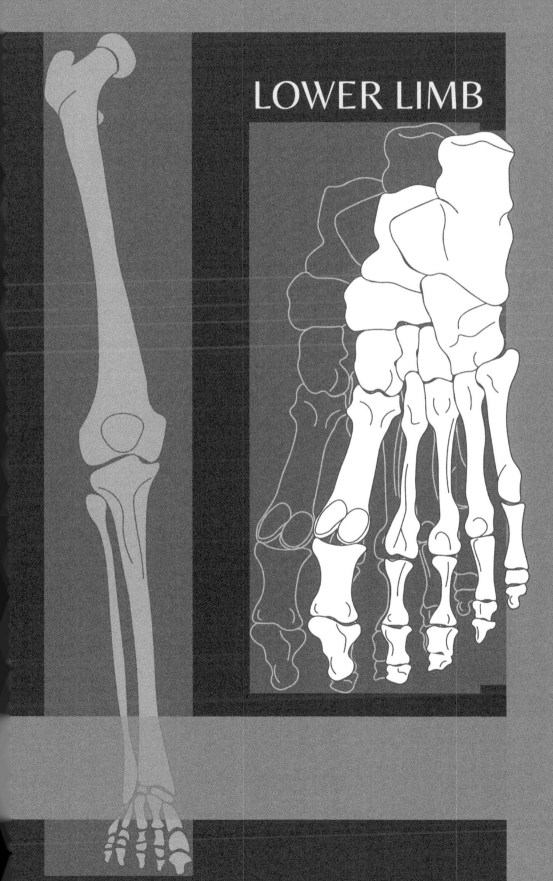

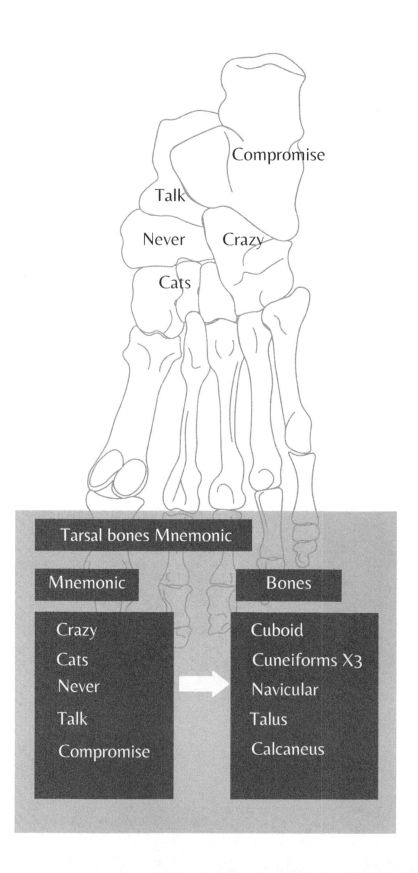

Compromise

Talk

Never   Crazy

Cats

Tarsal bones Mnemonic

Mnemonic	Bones
Crazy	Cuboid
Cats	Cuneiforms X3
Never	Navicular
Talk	Talus
Compromise	Calcaneus

Foot - Dosal & Plantar views

Dosal view

Plantar view

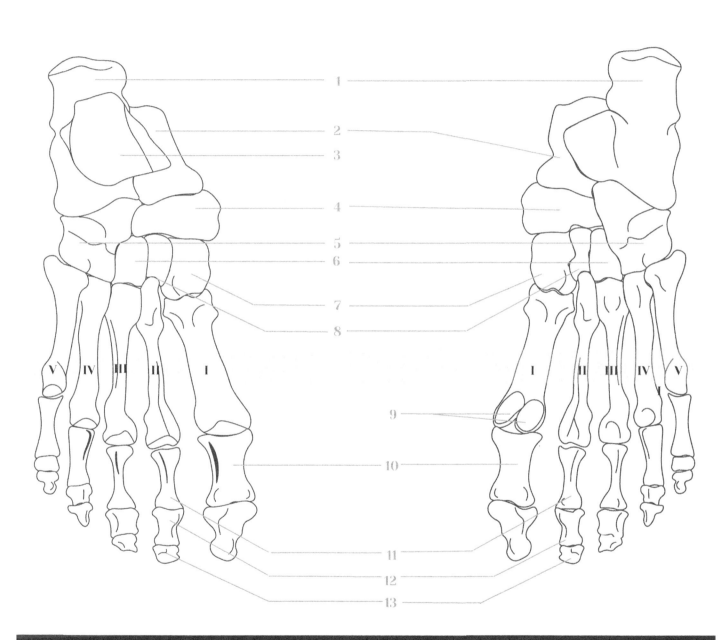

7 Tarsal Bones

- 1. Calcaneus
- 2. Talus Bone
- 3. Articular surface (Femur Bone)
- 4. Navicular bone
- 5. Cuboid Bone
- 6. Lateral cuneiform bone
- 7. Intermediate cuneiform bone
- 8. Medial cuneiform bone
- 9. Sesamoid bones
- (I) 1st Metatarsal bone
- (II) 2nd Metatarsal
- (III) 3rd Metatarsal
- (IV) 4th Metatarsal
- (V) 5th Metatarsal
- 10. Proximal phalanx (1st)
- 11. Proximal phalanx
- 12. Middle phalanx
- 13. Distal phalanx

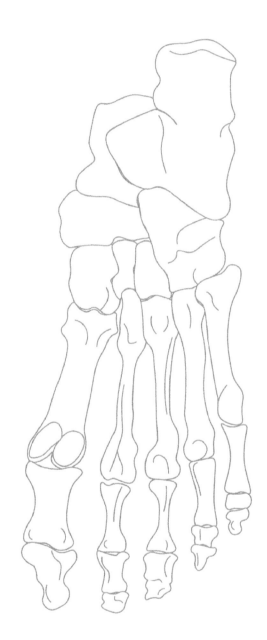

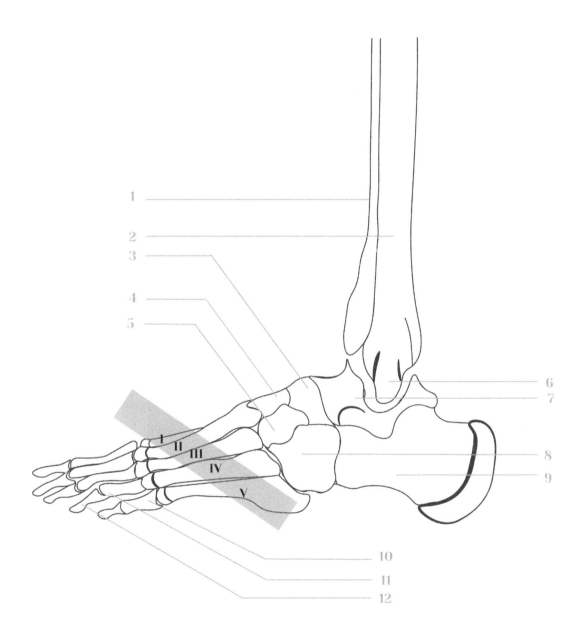

1
2
3
4
5
6
7
8
9
10
11
12

I
II
III
IV
V

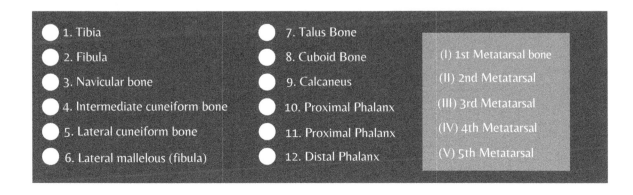

⚪ 1. Tibia	⚪ 7. Talus Bone
⚪ 2. Fibula	⚪ 8. Cuboid Bone
⚪ 3. Navicular bone	⚪ 9. Calcaneus
⚪ 4. Intermediate cuneiform bone	⚪ 10. Proximal Phalanx
⚪ 5. Lateral cuneiform bone	⚪ 11. Proximal Phalanx
⚪ 6. Lateral mallelous (fibula)	⚪ 12. Distal Phalanx

(I) 1st Metatarsal bone

(II) 2nd Metatarsal

(III) 3rd Metatarsal

(IV) 4th Metatarsal

(V) 5th Metatarsal

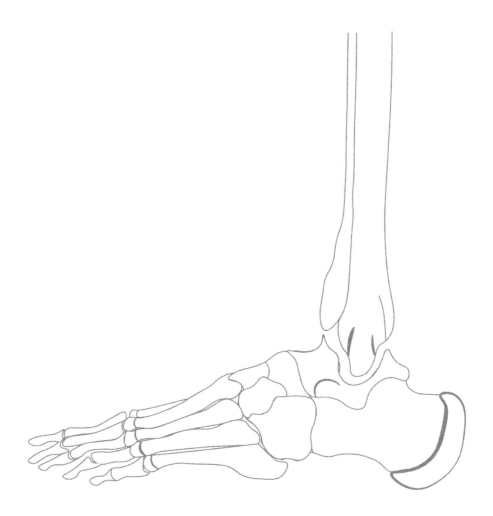

Leg - Anterior & Posterior views

Anterior view

Posterior view

1. Head (Femur)
2. Greater trochanter (Femur)
3. Neck (Femur)
4. Lesser trochanter (Femur)
5. Pectineal line
6. Femur (Shaft)
7. linea aspera
8. Lateral femoral condyle
9. Patella
10. Medial epycondyle
11. Medial femoral condyle
12. Intercondylar eminence
13. Tibial tuberosity
14. Tibia
15. Fibula
16. Lateral malleolus (Fibula)
17. Medial malleolus (Tibia)
18. Metatarsal bones
19. Proximal Phalanx (1st)
20. Distal Phalanx (1st)
21. Medial supracondylar line
21. Lateral supracondylar line
23. Talus (Tarsal bone)
24. Calcaneus (Tarsal bone)

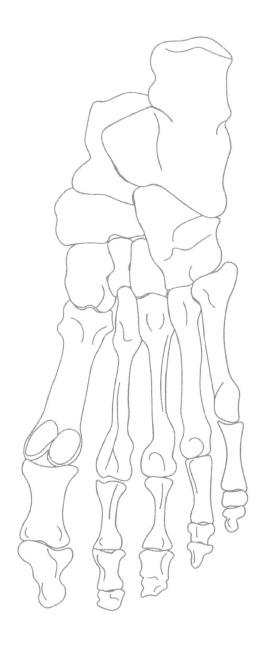

Leg and Proximal Femur

Proximal Femur (Posterior view)

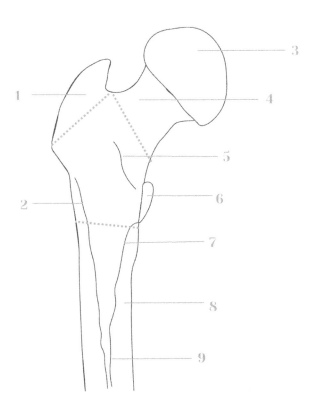

Leg (Anterolateral view)

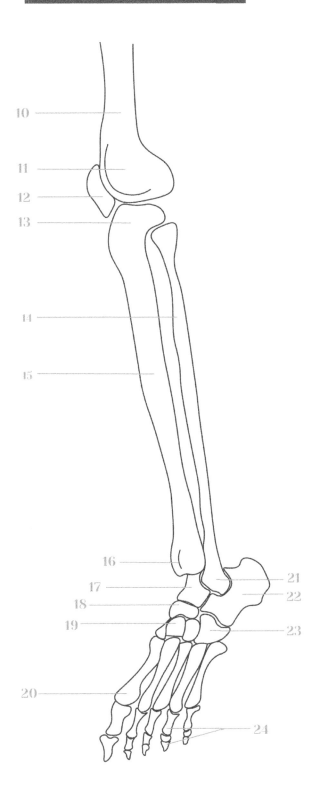

Proximal Femur (posterior view)	Leg (anterolateral view)
1. Greater trochanter	10. Distal Shaft (Femur)
2. Gluteal tuberosity	11. Lateral condyle of femur
3. Head (Femur)	12. Patela
4. Neck (Femur)	13. Lateral condyle of tibia
5. Intertrochanteric line	14. Fibula
6. Lesser trochanter	15. Tibia
7. Pectineal line	16. Medial malleolous (Tibia)
8. Shaft (Femur)	17. Talus
9. Linea Aspera	18. Navicular
	19. Cuneiform bone
	20. Metatarsal bone
	21. Lateral malleolous (Fibula)
	22. Calcaneus
	23. Cuboid
	24. Phalanges

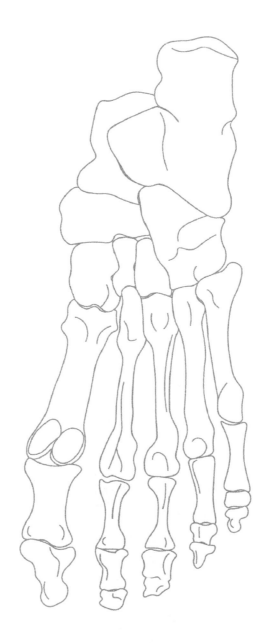

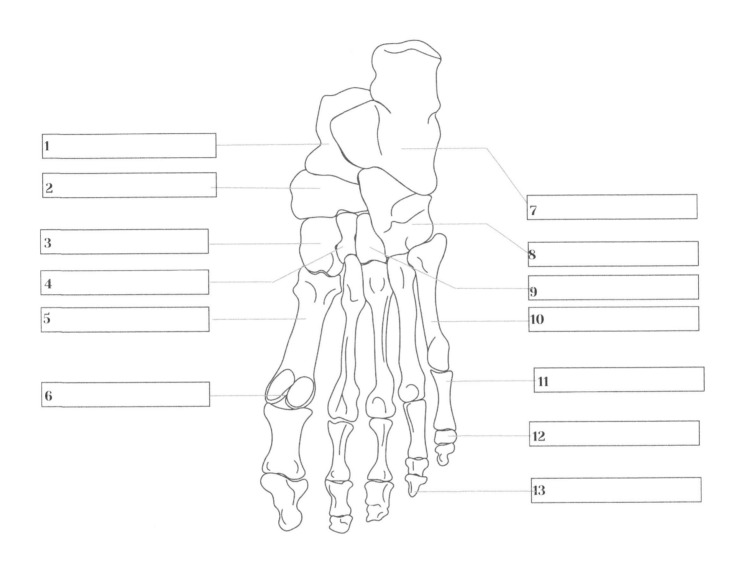

1

2

3

4

5

6

7

8

9

10

11

12

13

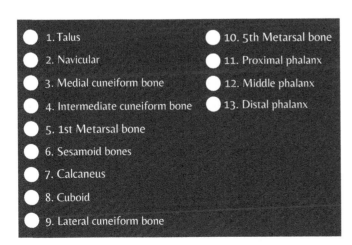

1. Talus
2. Navicular
3. Medial cuneiform bone
4. Intermediate cuneiform bone
5. 1st Metarsal bone
6. Sesamoid bones
7. Calcaneus
8. Cuboid
9. Lateral cuneiform bone
10. 5th Metarsal bone
11. Proximal phalanx
12. Middle phalanx
13. Distal phalanx

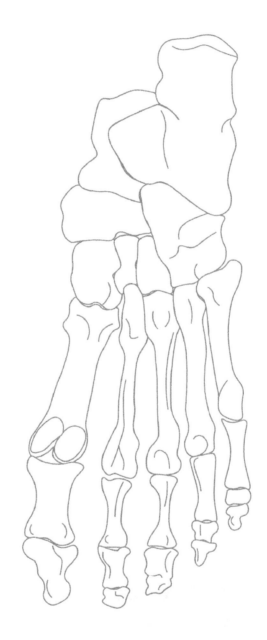

CHAPTER VI

VERTEBRAL COLUMN

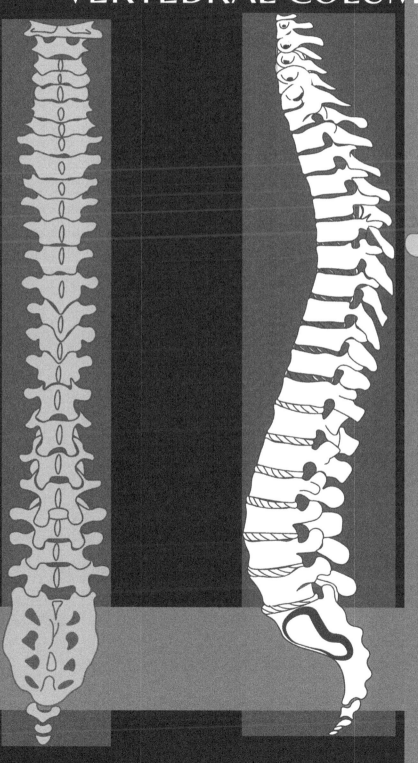

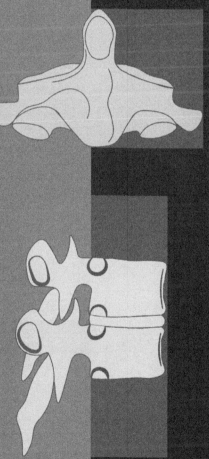

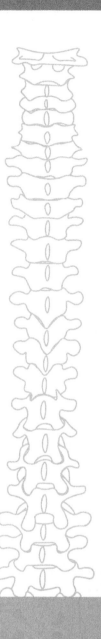

The Vertebral column

-Cervical Spine C1-C2

-Thoracic Spine T1-T12

-Lumbar Spine L1-L5

-Sacrum S1-S5 (Fused)

-Coccyx Co1-Co4 (Fused)

Kyphotic curves are primary curvatures that present during fetal development.

Lordotic Curves are secondary curvatures that develop post delivery.

Vertebral Column & Its Natural Curvatures

Vertebral column (Posterior view)

Curvatures (lateral view)

CERVICAL

THORACIC

LUMBAR

SACRAL & COCCYXGEAL

1

2

3

4

5

- 1. Cervical Curvature (Cervical lordosis)
- 2. Thoracic curvature (Thoracic kyphosis)
- 3. Lumbar curvature (Lumbar lordosis)
- 4. Sacrococcyxgeal curvature (Sacrococcyxgeal kyphosis)
- 5. Coccyx bone

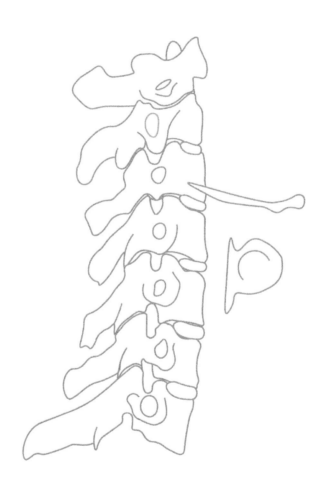

Cervical Vertebrae

Cervical spine (Lateral view)

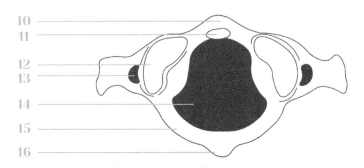

C1 -Atlas (Superior view)

C2 -Axis (Anterior view)

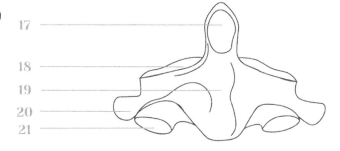

Cervical vertebra (Superior view)

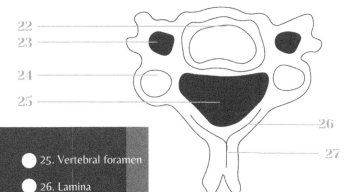

1. Posterior tubercle (C1-Atlas)
2. Spinous processes (C2-C4)
3. Lamina (C5)
4. Spinous process
5. Anterior tubercle (C1-Atlas)
6. Vertebral body (C2)
7. Hyoid bone
8. Thyroid cartilage
9. Transverse Process (C7)

C1 -Atlas (Superior view)

10. Anterior tubercle
11. Odontoid facet
12. Superior articular facet
13. Foramen transversarium

14. Vertebral foramen
15. Posterior arch
16. Posterior tubercle

C2 -Axis (Anterior view)

17. Odontoid process (Dens)
18. Superior articular facet
19. Vertebral body (C3)
20. Transverse process
21. Inferior articular process and facet

Cervical vertebra (Superior view)

22. Vertebral body (C3)
23. Foramen transversarium
24. Superior articular facet

25. Vertebral foramen
26. Lamina
27. Spinous process (bifurcated)

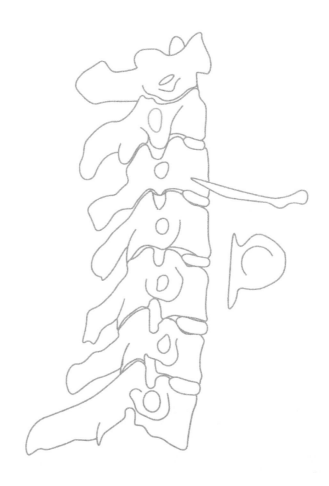

Thoracic vertebrae

Thoracic spine (Lateral view T1-T12)

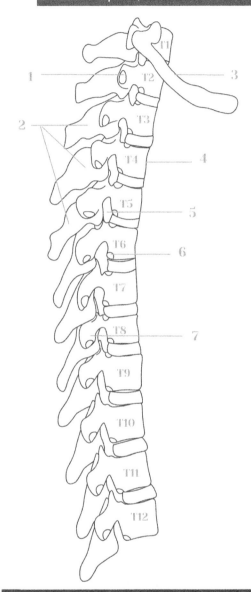

Thoracic vertebra (Superior view)

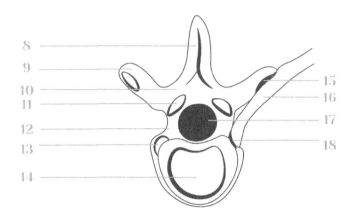

Thoracic vertebrae (Lateral view)

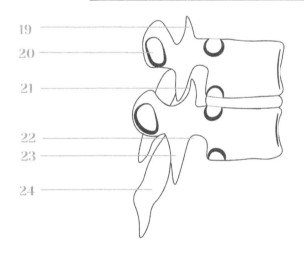

Thoracic spine (Lateral view T1-T9)

1. Rib facet (T2)
2. Spinous processes (T3-T5)
3. 1st Rib
4. Vertebral body (T4)
5. Intervetebral foramen
6. Rib facet (T6)
7. Transverse Process (T8)

12. Pedicle
13. Rib facet
14. Vertebral body
15. Costotransverse joint
16. Neck of Rib
17. Vertebral foramen
18. Costovertebral joint

23. Inferior articular process
24. Spinous process

Thoracic vertebra (Superior view)

8. Spinous process
9. Transverse Process
10. Lamina
11. Superior articular facet

Thoracic vertebrae (Lateral view)

19. Superior articular facet
20. Rib facet
21. Zygopophyseal joint
22. Inferior vertebral notch

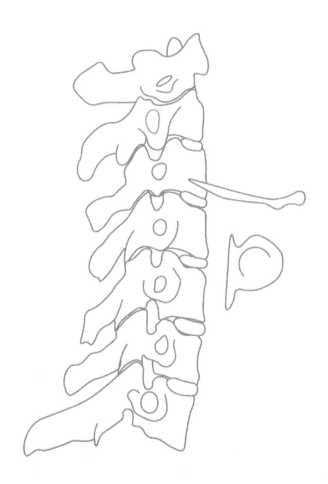

Lumbar Vertebra & Sacrum

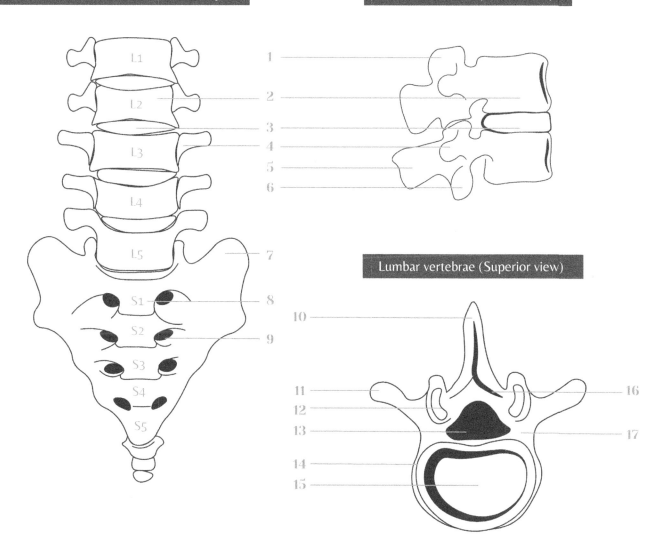

Lumbar vertebrae, Sacrum, and Coccyx

Lumbar vertebrae (Lateral view)

Lumbar vertebrae (Superior view)

LUMBAR VETEBRAE

SACRAL VETEBRAE

COCCYX

1. Superior articular process and facet
2. Vertebral body
3. Intervertebral disc
4. Transverse Process
5. Spinous process
6. Inferior articular process and facet
7. Ala of sacrum
8. Sacral body
9. Sacral foramen
10. Spinous process
11. Transverse Process
12. Superior articular process and facet
13. Vertebral foramen
15. Vertebral body
16. Lamina
17. Pedicle

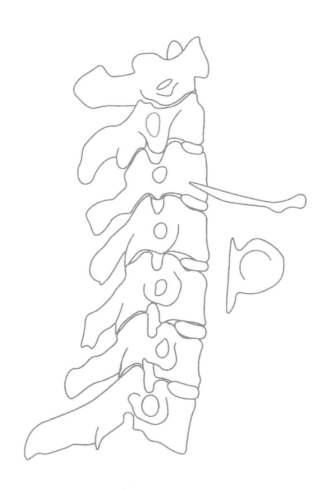

Vertebral Column - Review

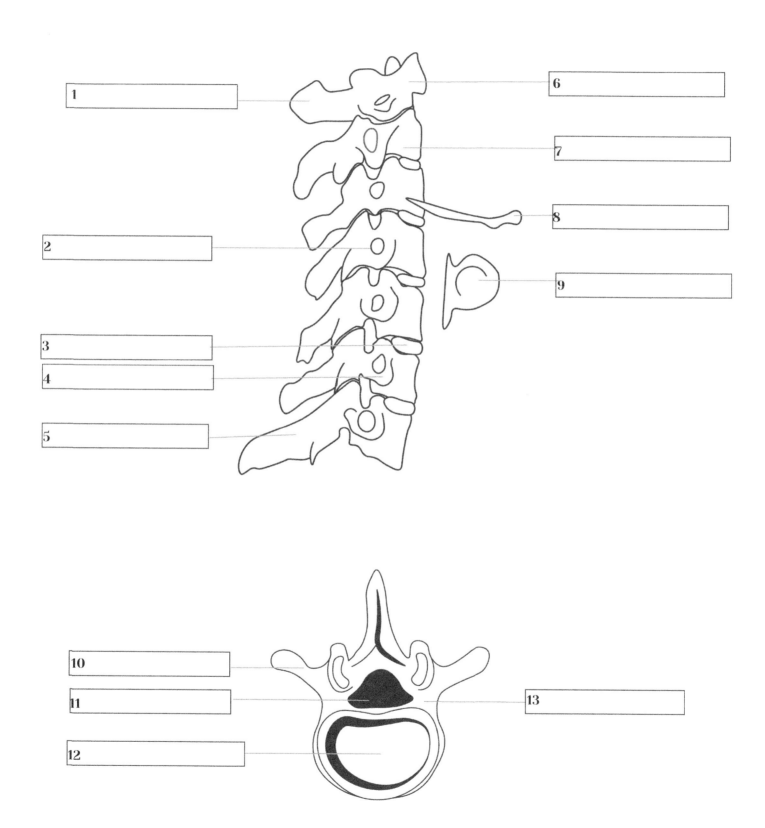

1

2

3

4

5

6

7

8

9

10

11

12

13

CHAPTER VII

PELVIC GIRDLE

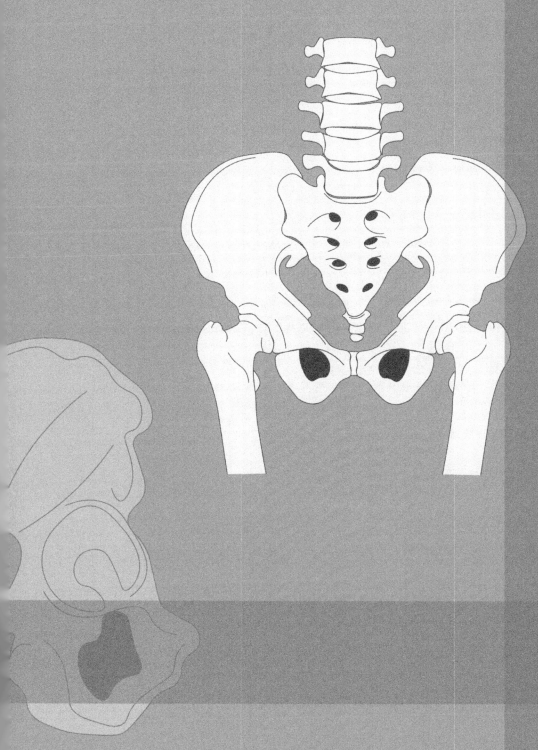

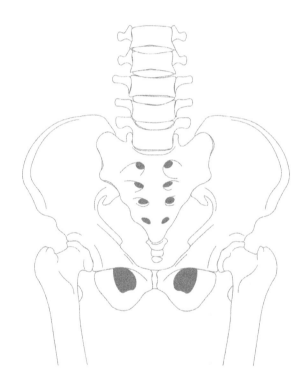

Pelvis with Lumbar Vertebrae

(Anterior view)

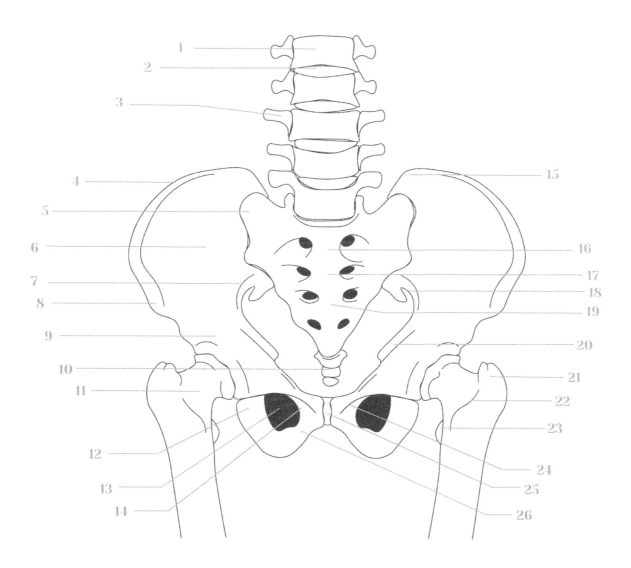

● 1. Vertebral body (L1)	● 10. Coccyx	● 19. 4th Sacral vertebra
● 2. Intervertebral disc	● 11. Neck (Femur)	● 20. Ischial spine
● 3. Transverse process (L3)	● 12. Ramus of Ischium	● 21. Greater trochanter (Femur)
● 4. Iliac crest	● 13. Obuturator foramen	● 22. Intertrochanteric line (Femur)
● 5. Ala of sacrum	● 14. Superior ramus of pubis	● 23. Lesser trochanter (Femur)
● 6. Iliac fossa	● 15. Posterior superior illiac spine	● 24. Pubic tubercle
● 7. Arcuate line (ilium)	● 16. 2nd Sacral vertebra	● 25. Pubic symphysis
● 8. Anterior superior illiac spine	● 17. 3rd Sacral vertebra	● 26. Inferior ramus of pubis
● 9. Iliopectineal eminence (Ilium)	● 18. Greater sciatic notch	

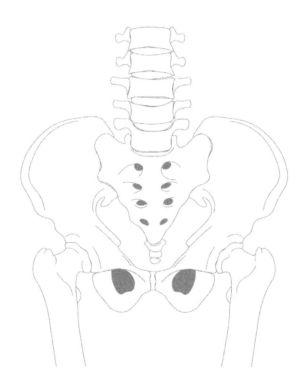

(Posterior view)

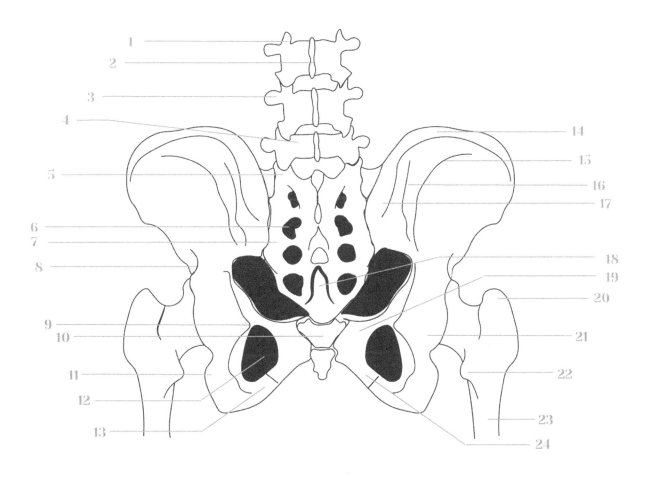

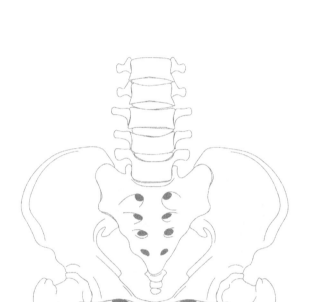

Hip bone - Lateral view

Right Hip / Coxal bone (Lateral view)

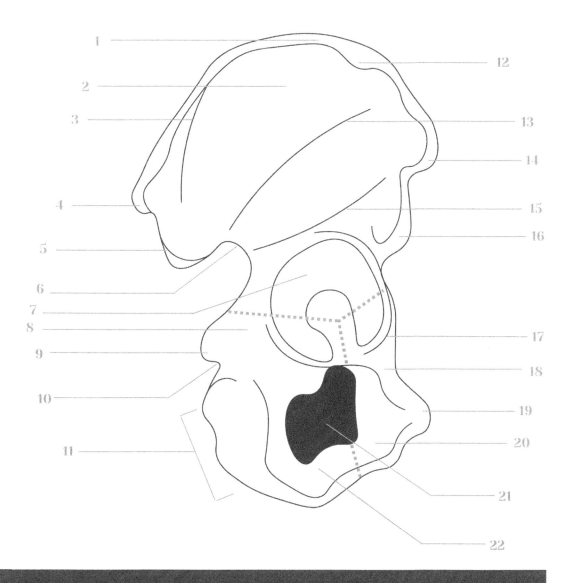

1. Iliac crest	10. Lesser sciatic notch	19. Pubic tubercle
2. Ala	11. Ischial tuberosity	20. Inferior ramus of pubis
3. Posterior gluteal line	12. Iliac tubercle	21. Obuturator foramen
4. Posterior superior iliac spine	13. Anterior gluteal line	22. Ramus of Ischium
5. Posterior inferior iliac spine	14. Anterior superior iliac spine	
6. Greater sciatic notch	15. Inferior gluteal line	
7. Acetabulum	16. Anterior inferior iliac spine	
8. Ischial body	17. Body of pubis	
9. Spine of ischium	18. Superior ramus of pubis	

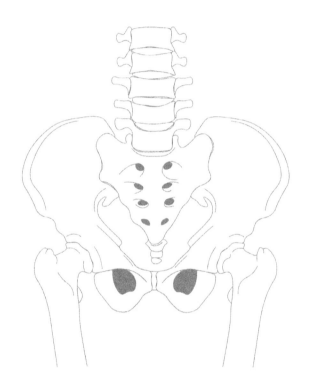

Pelvis - Review

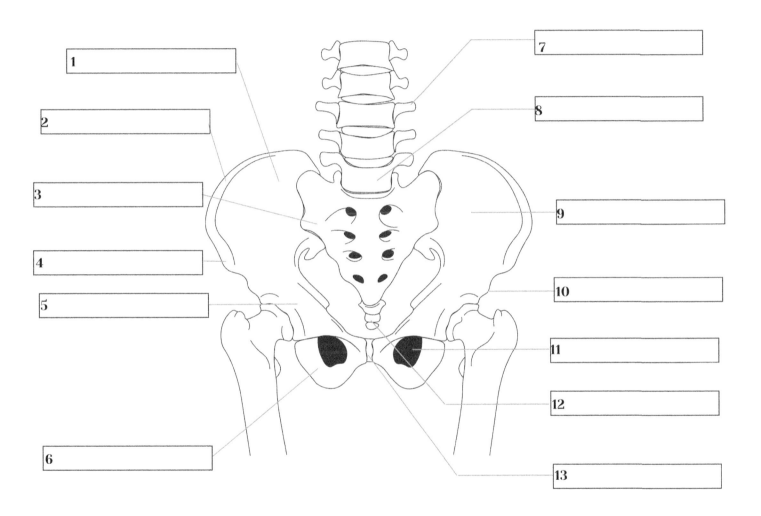

1

2

3

4

5

6

7

8

9

10

11

12

13

OTHER BOOKS FROM THE MEDICAL NOTES SERIES

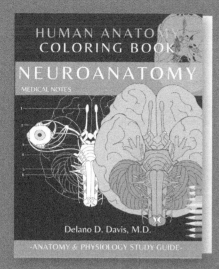

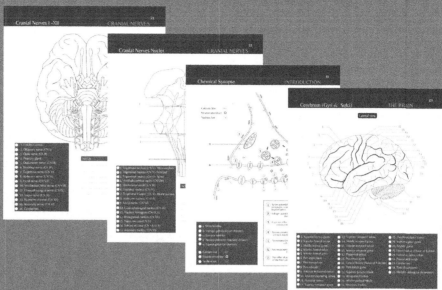

- Detailed neuroanatomical diagrams
- Gross anatomy & physiology
- High yield summaries and overviews
- Add & personalize your notes
- Chapter reviews and self-tests
- Access to video tutorials & quizzes

Scan QR code
to purchase ➡

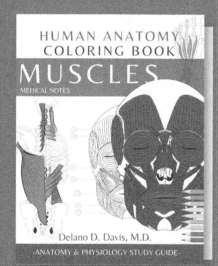

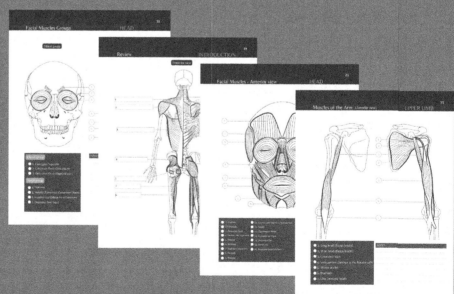

- Detailed diagrams of the muscles of the musculoskeletal system
- High yield summaries and overviews
- Facial muscle groups
- Upper limb & lower limb muscles
- Add & personalize your notes
- Access to video tutorial & quizzes

Scan QR code ➡
to purchase

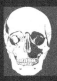

MEDICAL ESSENTIALS +

MEDICAL EDUCATION THE EASY WAY

Connect with us:

Follow us on all our social media platforms

MEDICAL ESSENTIALS PLUS

For questions and customer service;

Please leave a review of this book and send us an email at medicalessentialsplus@gmail.com
Follow Us on Instagram @ medicalessentialsplus
Subscribe to our Youtube channel " Medical Essentials Plus"
for tutorials and Quizzes.

Made in the USA
Las Vegas, NV
03 March 2024

86673356R00057